September 2007

Dear Jill,

with fond memories of our working together!

Warmly,

Susanne

Studienreihe

Psychologische Forschungsergebnisse

Band 128

ISSN 1435-666X

Verlag Dr. Kovač

Susanne Hörz

A Prototype of Borderline Personality Organization

Assessed by the Structured Interview of Personality Organization (STIPO)

Dear Jill,
warmest wishes
from
Susanne

Verlag Dr. Kovač

Hamburg
2007

VERLAG DR. KOVAČ
FACHVERLAG FÜR WISSENSCHAFTLICHE LITERATUR

Leverkusenstr. 13 · 22761 Hamburg · Tel. 040 - 39 88 80-0 · Fax 040 - 39 88 80-55

E-Mail info@verlagdrkovac.de · Internet www.verlagdrkovac.de

Bibliografische Information der Deutschen Nationalbibliothek
Die Deutsche Nationalbibliothek verzeichnet diese Publikation
in der Deutschen Nationalbibliografie;
detaillierte bibliografische Daten sind im Internet
über http://dnb.d-nb.de abrufbar.

ISSN: 1435-666X

ISBN: 978-3-8300-2762-1

Zugl.: Dissertation, Ludwig-Maximilians-Universität München, 2006

Gedruckt auf holz-, chlor- und säurefreiem Papier Alster Digital. Alster Digital ist alterungsbeständig und erfüllt die Normen für Archivbeständigkeit ANSI 3948 und ISO 9706.

Acknowledgments

I would like to thank the many people who have contributed to this book. First of all, I am very grateful to my doctoral advisors from both sides of the Atlantic for their excellent mentorship: Professor Wolfgang Mertens at the Ludwig-Maximilians-Universität München and Professor John Clarkin at the Personality Disorders Institute, Weill Medical College of Cornell University.

This study is the result of a cooperation between the Department of Psychology of Ludwig-Maximilians-Universität München and the Personality Disorders Institute of Weill Medical College of Cornell University. I feel fortunate for the opportunity to have worked at the Personality Disorders Institute with Professor Otto Kernberg, who shaped this dissertation through his insights and knowledge. Professors Eve Caligor and Barry Stern guided me in the development of my research project, taught me about the STIPO and greatly impacted my study.

I appreciate the collaboration with the other members and staff of the Personality Disorders Institute, especially Drs. Frank Yeomans and Jorge Cassab, and Drs. Ann Appelbaum, Ken Critchfield, Jill Delaney, Diana Diamond, Pamela Foelsch, Kay Haran, James Hull, Paulina Kernberg, Kenneth Levy, Armand Loranger, Larry Rockland, and Michael Stone. I am grateful for the openness and help of Dr. Nudman and the staff of Unit 5 North at the Westchester Division of New York Presbyterian Hospital who enabled me to be part of the unit and helped organize the interviews. I also wish to thank the many individuals who participated in the study and went through extensive interviews.

I am indebted to my colleagues and the associates of the Munich TFP-Institute, whose support and interest has contributed largely to the finalization of this dissertation. In particular, I owe my special thanks to Professor Peter Buchheim, and to Dr. Claudia Bailer, Professor Cord Benecke, Dr. Anna Buchheim, Professor Stefan Doering, Professor Hans Förstl, Dipl.-Psych. Petra Holler, Dr. Mathias Lohmer, Dr. Philipp Martius, Dr. Michael Rentrop, Dr. Agnes Schneider-Lehmann, Professor Almuth Sellschopp, Flora Gräfin von Spreti and Wilhelm Graf von Spreti.

This study was awarded the "Hamburger Fellowship Persönlichkeitsstörungen 2006" by the Gesellschaft zur Erforschung und Therapie von Persönlichkeitsstörungen (GePs) e.V. and the LBK Hamburg GmbH.

This dissertation was supported by grants from "HWP– Hochschul- und Wissenschaftsprogramm zur Förderung der Chancengleichheit für Frauen in Forschung und Lehre" to Susanne Hörz, for which I am grateful. I wish to express special thanks to Professor Ulla Mitzdorf of the LMU München. This program is an agreement between the federal government of Germany and the federal states and was allocated by the Frauenbeauftragte der LMU München. The overall study was supported by grants from the International Psychoanalytic Association (primary investigator Barry L. Stern).

Finally, my parents receive my deepest gratitude for their love and the many years of support during my studies that provided the foundation for this work. I wish to dedicate this thesis to the memory of my father, Wolfram Hörz.

Table of Contents

List of Tables

List of Figures

Abbreviations

PD	Personality Disorder
BPD	Borderline Personality Disorder
BPO	Borderline Personality Organization
NPO	Neurotic Personality Organization
PPO	Psychotic Personality Organization
STIPO	Structured Interview of Personality Organization (Clarkin, Caligor, Stern & Kernberg, 2004)
IPO	Inventory of Personality Organization (Clarkin, Foelsch & Kernberg, 2001)
SNAP	Schedule of Nonadaptive and Adaptive Personality (Clark, 1993)
IIP-PD	Inventory of Interpersonal Problems, Personality Disorders Scales (Pilkonis et al., 1996)
BFI-44	Big Five Inventory –44 (John, Donahue & Kentle, 1991)
PANAS	Positive Affect Negative Affect Scale (Watson, Clark & Harkness, 1994)
BDI	Buss- Durkee-Inventory (Buss & Durkee, 1957)
BSI	Brief Symptom Inventory (Derogatis, 1993)
M, SD, N, Min, Max	Mean, Standard Deviation, Sample Size, Minimum, Maximum

I INTRODUCTION

"I don't like being alone – when I am alone, I feel insecure, I don't know who I am anymore. Sometimes I go to a shop and speak to the salesperson – if that person speaks to me, I know I still exist. This is how I often try to get a sense of who I am."

"When I look at pictures from four years ago, I cannot believe that that is the same person I am now. I cannot understand what I thought or felt a year ago, I cannot imagine that person and I have anything in common…"

"In romantic relationships I lose myself. I turn into the person my boyfriend wants me to be. Finally I believe I am that person. I want to stay the same but I cannot…"

"When my partner and I broke up he told me I always accused him of doing things I was doing myself, like being jealous and suspicious. I am sure he is wrong."

"My friend? Oh, she is the best friend you can imagine. She is friendly, thoughtful, concerned about me. But often she is also the most selfish person I know."

"I hate it when my best friend goes on vacation. Usually this is the time when I start looking for a new best friend. She is thoughtless to leave me without calling more often. I really have no idea what she thinks about me."

These are statements patients made in the *Structured Interview of Personality Organization* (Clarkin et al., 2004). Clinicians and researchers encounter many versions of these complaints with different patients, but they all describe similar difficulties. Several areas can be identified in which these individuals may have problems: in the interaction with other people, in perception of self and others, in aggression towards self and others and in use of more primitive defense operations. These patients most often are diagnosed with personality disorders, and thorough diagnosis frequently shows that they are located at the level of Borderline Personality Organization.

In this study, the diagnosis of patients with personality disorders will be investigated. After a brief overview of personality disorders, and the diagnosis of personality disorders according to the Diagnostic and Statistical Manual of Mental Disorders (DSM-IV; American Psychiatric Association, 1994). The foundation of this study, Otto Kernberg's main concepts of Borderline Personality Organization (BPO), will be introduced. Then, several methods for the diagnosis of personality disorders will be described and a new interview, the *Structured Interview of Personality Organization* (STIPO), developed by Clarkin, Caligor, Stern and Kernberg (2004) will be presented.

In the present research project, the STIPO and several instruments assessing different aspects of personality and temperament were administered to a clinical sample. The core question of this study was: when diagnosed using the STIPO, what do all patients located at borderline personality organization have in common? Can certain areas be identified in which these patients show the same deficits and which differentiate them from other higher structured patient groups? To answer these questions, experts on Kernberg's theory of personality organization formed a consensus of which STIPO domains would best demonstrate these common deficits in borderline patients. This expert consensus was called a "prototype of Borderline Personality Organization". By comparing the STIPO results of the clinical sample to the prototypical profile, a similarity index was established which reflected each individual's similarity to the prototype.

In part, this methodology replicated a procedure developed by Miller and colleagues (2001) and used by Trull and colleagues (2003) in which they tested the hypothesis that Borderline Personality Disorder (BPD) is a maladaptive variant of personality traits included within the five-factor model (FFM) of personality. This model emphasizes the five personality domains neuroticism, extraversion, openness to experience, agreeableness, and conscientiousness, and their usefulness in explaining personality disorders. Based on expert-consensus ratings of five-factor model facets, Trull and colleagues developed a prototype for BPD. They computed a similarity index by correlating the expert prototypical profile with each individual's ratings from an instrument operationalizing the FFM (NEO-PI-R; Costa & McCrae, 1992b), indicating the individual's similarity to the prototypical FFM profile.

The methodology used in this study was similar. A STIPO-based prototypical profile was generated by experts on Borderline Personality Organization and the STIPO data obtained from a sample of patients with and without personality disorders was used to compare each patient to the theoretical prototypic profile. Given the atheoretical origins of the FFM, a model originally designed for the explanation of normal personality but that has nevertheless been found to explain considerable variation in the personality disorder, testing a prototype based on the STIPO was expected to prove valuable; as the STIPO was designed specifically to test a theory of personality organization closely related to personality disorder and health.

The STIPO derived prototype of BPO was tested in several respects. First, its ability to differentiate between clinically relevant patient groups within the sample was examined. Different patient clusters, grouped according to their similarity to the prototype, were analyzed regarding meaningful differences in general functioning and symptoms of axis I and II pathology.

Next, the BPO similarity index was examined in relation to a set of self-report measures in order to assess its convergent validity and incremental validity. For convergent validity, self-report measures assessing different aspects of personality and temperament were employed which were expected to be associated to the STIPO domains (e.g. traits like mistrust, entitlement, aggression as well as negative temperament, interpersonal difficulties like interpersonal sensitivity and various aspects of hostility). The relationship of variables expected not to correlate highly with the BPO index were examined, such as positive temperament or joviality. For incremental validity, the ability of the prototypical domains to explain variance over the dimensions of the FFM and also the self-report precursor of the STIPO (IPO; Foelsch et al., 2000) was tested.

In the final part of this study, with the goal of exemplifying the use of the STIPO and testing the usefulness of the prototype, the results of four patients from separate patient groups who differed in their similarity to the prototype were analyzed in detail. Four patients located at different levels of personality organization were chosen to show how the STIPO and the BPO prototype discriminate between these levels. Furthermore, the results from the STIPO and self-report measures are shown in context with their present life situation and described in detail.

Overall, the development and validation of the STIPO and the BPO prototype are expected to give important insights into the diagnosis of personality disorders based on a psychoanalytic theory. The goal is to help clinicians and researchers to focus on the most important aspects when diagnosing patients with personality disorders using an instrument like the STIPO.

II THEORETICAL AND EMPIRICAL BACKGROUND

1 Personality disorders

In this chapter personality disorders will be introduced as described in the *Diagnostic and Statistical Manual of Mental Disorders* (DSM-IV; American Psychiatric Association, 1994) and a brief historical overview of the scientific study of personality disorders will be presented. Also, controversies about the DSM multiaxial assessment and the conceptualization of personality disorders according to categorical versus dimensional models will be summarized.

Personality disorders are a group of mental disturbances defined by the fourth edition of the DSM (APA, 1994) as enduring patterns of inner experience and behavior that deviate markedly from the expectations of the culture of the individual who exhibits it. These patterns are inflexible and pervasive across many situations. The onset of the patterns can be traced back at least to the beginning of adulthood. To be diagnosed as a personality disorder, a behavioral pattern must cause significant distress or impairment in personal, social, or occupational situations.

History

This contemporary definition of personality disorders taken from the DSM system was preceded by other approaches to personality disorders which date back at least to the 19th century. Pinel (1809) established the scientific study of abnormal personalities. With his "Manie sans délire" he described individuals with disturbances of affective functions but unimpaired cognitive abilities. His model of the origin of individual reaction patterns, that is the combined influence of upbringing, interactions and individual history with a genetic predisposition, has remained important in today's etiological concepts of personality disorders. In 1891, Koch described individuals who showed moral insanity, which was the predominant form of personality disorder throughout the 19th century, as "psychopathic". Later on, German psychiatry made a clear distinction between psychopathic personality and neurosis, on the one hand, and psychosis on the other. Schneider (1950) coined the definition of psychopathic personalities as "abnormal personalities who either suffer personally because of their abnormality or make a community suffer because of it". He provided a classification of ten varieties of abnormal personality which are similar to the diagnoses in DSM-IV (APA; 1994) and the 10th revision of the *International Classification of Diseases* (ICD-10; World Health Organization, 1992).

The first psychoanalytic classifications of character pathology were given by Freud (1908; 1931) and by Abraham (1921). They described character pathology based on their understanding of instinctual, especially libidinal, motivations. The important psychoanalytic definitions of oral, anal, phallic or genital characters according to psychosexual development stages stem from these conceptualizations. The psychoanalyst Reich (1933) defined personality disorders – but also the development of "normal" character – as associated with use of characteristic defenses. His work on analysis of the patient's "character armor" was important for the psychoanalytic approach of personality disorders. Fenichel (1945) developed a typology of character disturbances which incorporated modifications of Freud's, Abraham's and Reich's work and which was one of the first extensive descriptions of character types.

In US-American psychiatry, the monograph "The Mask of Sanity" by Cleckley (1941) strongly influenced the contemporary concept of personality disorders. He advocated applying the term psychopathy narrowly only to individuals with antisocial behaviors which could not be explained through psychosis, neurosis or mental retardation. Nevertheless, in the first version of the DSM, "psychopathic personalities" described a broad array of disorders which had in common maladaptive behaviors and of which only one subgroup was named "antisocial" (Penna, 1981).

Nowadays, the differentiation between personality disorders and mental disorders is common in psychoanalytic terminology. Ermann (2004) states that the term "neurosis" is employed very broadly and should be clearly used to define a disorder which is based on a neurotic development. He distinguishes between two groups of neurotic disorders: first, mental disorders with functional impairment and symptoms (e.g. depression, anxiety disorders and dissociative disorders), which are usually caused by neurotic conflicts. Second, personality disorders with character pathology, at different structural levels. Regarding the differences in terminologies, it should be noted that in the chapters referring to Kernberg's classification system, the term neurotic personality organization comprises both symptomatic neuroses and neurotic character pathology, the latter being personality disorders at the level of neurotic personality (Kernberg, 1984).

Personality disorders in the DSM system

In the first version of the DSM (American Psychiatric Association, 1952), personality disorders were introduced as a broad category of disorders with five subclasses, personality pattern disturbances, personality trait disturbances, sociopathic personality disturbances, special symptom reactions, and transient situational personality disorders. The diagnosis of a personality disorder could be given alternatively or in addition to other mental disorders. After the criticism had been raised that clinicians needed to choose between a "neurotic condition" and a personality disorder when both appeared to be present (Ward et al., 1962), the placement of personality disorders on a separate axis with DSM-III (APA) in 1980 was welcomed. With DSM-III, the psychodynamic view was abandoned and replaced by a behavioral model. DSM became atheoretical, provided classifications of the disorders, which were based mainly on clinical descriptions, and introduced the multiaxial system which is still in practice today. It consists of five axes: axis I disorders are conceptualized as mental illnesses, which have an onset throughout adult life, are episodic, and are distinguishable from normal personality functioning. On axis II, personality disorders and also forms of mental retardation are described which persist for a long time and usually commence in adolescence (note that in the further text the term "axis II" will be used to refer only to the personality disorders and not to the specific developmental disorders also located on this axis). On axis III, physical conditions are coded which play a role in the development, continuance, or exacerbation of axis I and II disorders. Axis IV indicates the severity of psychosocial stressors, and on axis V, the highest level of functioning is rated. Since DSM-III, clinicians were encouraged to diagnose personality disorders along with other mental disorders (Frances, 1980), and research suggests that since this division the recognition of personality disorders in clinical practice has increased (Blashfield & McElroy, 1987; Loranger, 1990).

Clusters of personality disorders

The widely used DSM classification system (APA, 1994) describes three clusters of personality disorders. All personality disorders have in common inflexible and enduring patterns of cognition, affect and behavior that cause clinically significant distress in different areas of functioning. The personality disorders are grouped into clusters according to their prominent characteristics (compare table 1). Cluster A, the “odd cluster”, includes disorders marked by odd or eccentric behaviors, namely paranoid, schizoid and schizotypal personality disorders. Patients with these disorders exhibit strange or eccentric behaviors. Cluster B disorders are characterized by dramatic, emotional or erratic behaviors, including antisocial, borderline, histrionic and narcissistic personality disorders. Finally, cluster C disorders are characterized by anxious or fearful behaviors and consist of avoidant, dependent and obsessive compulsive personality disorders. The cluster structure of personality disorders has been confirmed in several studies (e.g. Kass et al., 1985; Sanislow et al., 2002).

Table 1. The three clusters of personality disorders according to the DSM-IV (APA, 1994)

Cluster A	**Cluster B**	**Cluster C**
Paranoid PD	Antisocial PD	Avoidant PD
Schizoid PD	Borderline PD	Dependent PD
Schizotypal PD	Histrionic PD	Obsessive-Compulsive PD
	Narcissistic PD	

Heterogeneity

In the DSM system, the diagnosis of a specific personality disorder is given in a polythetic format, requiring a certain number of fulfilled criteria to assign a specific diagnosis (for example, any 5 out of 9). The criteria consist of behaviors which are considered typical for the specific personality disorder. Although the introduction of fixed and explicit diagnostic criteria through DSM-III has lead to improved interrater reliability and standardization of diagnostic criteria (Kendall, 1982; Spitzer, Forman & Nee, 1979), several aspects of this diagnostic method have been criticized. Widiger and colleagues (1984) state that the diagnostic efficiency of the DSM could be improved by applying principles of actuarial decision theory, for example by developing methods for weighting the diagnostic criteria differentially, rather than assuming that all criteria are equally important.

The polythetic format of criteria might be consistent with clinical reality, but also results in strong heterogeneity: Two individuals might be assigned the same diagnosis albeit fulfilling very different criteria. Clarkin et al. (1983) indicated that there were 93 different ways a person could meet the DSM-III (and DSM-III-R) polythetic diagnostic criteria for BPD (i.e., any combination of 5 of 8, 6 of 8, 7 of 8, or 8 of 8 diagnostic criteria). DSM-IV added an additional diagnostic criterion without changing the threshold for the diagnosis, contributing to even further heterogeneity. There are now 151 different ways of meeting the DSM-IV criteria for BPD.

Co-occurrence of personality disorders

Diagnostic overlap is present because some criteria appear in several of the different personality disorders. For example, items assessing the same trait are part of several diagnoses: one of the criteria in the description of schizotypal personality disorder is social isolation, a criterion portraying schizoid personality disorder is the lack of close friendships and avoidant personality disorders show "social withdrawal". Thus, these categories lack distinctiveness (Livesley, 1985). Furthermore, a large number of patients (in the range of 21-49%) who meet the DSM *general* criteria for a personality disorder, do not meet the required amount of criteria for any *specific* category (Verheul & Widiger, 2004). These patients are classified as "personality disorder, not otherwise specified", emphasizing the importance of also taking the overall definition of personality pathology into account, not only the categorical disorder-specific assessment. Furthermore, patients often fulfill criteria of different personality disorders, thus being assigned several diagnoses. This comorbidity, or co-occurrence of several personality disorders in one individual has often been reported both in clinical samples (Oldham et al., 1992; Pilkonis et al., 1995; Zimmerman, Rothschild & Chelminski, 2005) as well in nonclinical samples (Watson & Sinha, 1998). For example, Herpertz and colleagues (1994) found that 41% patients of a clinical sample had more than one personality disorder according to DSM-III-R criteria. Nurnberg et al. (1991) found that 82% of patients with BPD who were part of an outpatient sample had at least one additional personality disorder, which was not confined to any one of the three designated axis II clusters.

Comorbidity with axis I disorders

Comorbidity of axis II disorders with axis I is also frequently found and makes the diagnostic assessment more difficult. As mentioned before, the two axes were separated to ensure that clinicians did not ignore relevant conditions like personality disorders which might be more easily overlooked as compared to the clinical disorders recorded on axis I. Westen and Shedler (2000) discuss several aspects regarding the distinction between axis I and II. For example, one of the concepts is that axis I disorders are considered states that could presumably remit, whereas axis II codes enduring traits. This distinction is likely to a certain degree, but for example does not apply to a psychotic patient's state becoming a trait over time. However, the distinction between the two axes has led to a large body of literature on comorbidity between the two axis. For example, McGlashan and colleagues (2000) found that patients in the "Collaborative Longitudinal Personality Disorders Study" diagnosed with personality disorders on average had 3.4 axis I lifetime diagnoses and 1.4 co-occurring personality disorders. In particular, patients with schizotypal or borderline personality disorder had more co-occurring disorders than patients with avoidant, obsessive-compulsive personality disorder or patients with Major Depression. An especially strong link emerged between avoidant personality disorder and social phobia, between BPD and Posttraumatic Stress Disorder and between BPD and substance use. The patterns of co-occuring diagnoses had been reported in previous studies as well (e.g. Dolan-Sewell, Krueger & Shea, 2001). The association of personality pathology with axis I symptoms has important implications for treatment outcome. Thus, several studies have shown that comorbid personality disorders indicate worse prognosis for patients with a variety of axis I disorders, for example for panic disorders (Noyes, Jr. et al., 1990) or for alcohol abuse (Verheul, van den & Hartgers, 1998).

Many aspects of how maladaptive personality traits and other mental disorders relate to one another have been discussed (Pfohl, 1999). First, personality disorders might predispose individuals to the development of a mental disorder (Johnson & Wonderlich, 1992). For example, a schizotypal personality disorder might be a predisposing factor for schizophrenia. Next, mental disorders might predispose the development of maladadaptive personality traits or a personality disorder. Also, personality pathology can alter the course or affect the treatment of mental disorders (Dolan-Sewell, Krueger, & Shea, 2001; Widiger & Seidlitz, 2002). And lastly, underlying variables or biological factors might predispose the development of both and show phenomenological overlap. An example is the phenomenological overlap between avoidant personality disorder and social phobia.

On the whole, as Westen and colleagues (2006) summarize, contemporary psychopathology research has shown that virtually all non-psychotic syndromes share common factors with other syndromes and that these factors comprise what is commonly understood as aspects of personality. For example, Krueger (1999) found underlying core psychopathological processes, that is two factors of internalizing versus externalizing problems, accounting for comorbidity results in a large sample. Also, Blatt (e.g. 1983; 2007) emphasizes that anaclitic (preoccupation with issues of interpersonal relatedness) and introjective (preoccupation with self-definition) personality dimensions are the basic core of most forms of psychopathology. The implication is that for a full understanding of the symptoms a person presents, it is important to examine his or her personality structure.

Dimensional assessment

Closely linked to the conclusion by Westen and colleagues (2006), and related to the categorical classification of personality disorders in the DSM system, an extensive discussion about alternative ways of assessing personality pathology and moving to a more dimensional assessment has emerged (e.g. Widiger & Frances, 1985; Widiger & Simonsen, 2005). Clark et al. (2005) suggest personality disorders might be considered as maladaptive personality traits of general personality functioning. The co-occurrence with disorders on axis I might also be explained by these common, underlying dimensions of maladaptive traits. Livesley (1998) proposes an empirically based classification of personality disorder, according to which personality disorders, conceptualized as mental disorders, should be classified as a single diagnostic entity on axis I along with other mental disorders. He suggests describing clinically significant personality traits on axis II. This way the classification would explicitly distinguish between the diagnosis of personality disorder and the assessment of personality on clinically relevant dimensions. Emphasizing the need for dimensional assessment, he suggests a list of 16 basic dispositional traits to describe personality disorder, and also three higher-order patterns: emotional dysregulation, dissocial behavior and inhibitedness. According to this model, personality disorders would be conceptualized not only on a continuum with axis I disorders, but also at the far spectrum of normal personality. Integrating the classification of personality disorders with dimensional models of general personality structure also would take into account a considerable amount of personality disorder symptomatology within the general population (Livesley, 2003).

Another well-known dimensional approach is the Five Factor Model (FFM) of general personality functioning which proposes to conceptualize personality disorders based on personality traits (Costa & McCrae, 1992a). The FFM of personality was derived lexically through studies of the English language to identify the domains of personality functioning which are the most important in describing the personality traits of oneself and other persons. It has emphasized five domains of personality, identified as neuroticism, extraversion, openness to experience, agreeableness and conscientiousness, each of which also can be divided into six underlying facets. In an attempt to explain personality pathology through the FFM, Widiger and colleagues have provided profiles of personality disorders described by the FFM facets (Widiger et al., 1994). Another approach of relating the FFM model to personality disorders was asking personality disorder researchers to explain prototypical personality disorders by FFM descriptors, which showed that the personality disorders could be described sufficiently in terms of the FFM facets (Lynam & Widiger, 2001; Miller et al., 2001; Samuel & Widiger, 2004). The validity of the FFM has been questioned by some authors (Benjamin, 1993; 1994a; 1994b; Block, 1995), in particular regarding the utility for clinicians. One concern is that as the five-factor model is derived from factor analysis of adjectives, these lists of adjectives may be inadequate for describing the complexities of personality. The language of the FFM also has been considered to be too superficial for clinical descriptions, that it is not differentiated enough for scientific and clinical purposes (e.g. Westen, 1995). Also, the ability of the FFM of discriminating between different personality disorders was not confirmed by Skodol et al. (2005). Having administered a FFM questionnaire to a large sample of patients, the results only indicated that the personality disordered patients could be distinguished from community norms on the personality dimensions of the FFM, but all shared the same extreme configuration of high Neuroticism, low Agreeableness, and low Conscientiousness. Put together, although the FFM is based on a dimensional approach and has proven some empirical validity, it could be criticized that it lacks a theoretical base and is only a descriptive model. The use of the FFM for diagnostic purposes as opposed to describing the personality disorders from the perspective of general personality pathology remains unclear.

Clinical implications

It has become clear that a multitude of conceptualizations for personality disorders exists. All the more, it is important to realize the impact of personality pathology on clinical routine. Patients with personality disorders are common in primary care settings and show extensive histories of psychiatric outpatient, inpatient, and psychopharmacologic treatment (Bender et al., 2001). The prevalence of personality disorders ranges from 20 to 50 % in clinical populations, depending on outpatient or inpatient status, the method of diagnosis and also on the country the sample was composed in. Merikangas and Weissman (1986) found that approximately half of those receiving mental health treatment also suffered from a personality disorder. Zimmermann, Rothschild and Chelminski (2005) found that 45.5% of a large psychiatric outpatient sample was diagnosed with a personality disorder (including "personality disorder not otherwise specified"). In a German inpatient sample, Herpertz, Steinmeyer and Sass (1994) found 20 to 30% diagnosed with personality disorders. In patients seeking admission to a German psychosomatic hospital, Fydrich and Schmitz (1996) found that 27% fulfilled criteria for a personality disorder. In the normal population, the prevalence of personality disorders is estimated between nine and 15 percent (Grant et al., 2004; Lenzenweger et al., 2007; Reich, Yates & Nduaguba, 1989; Torgersen, Kringlen & Cramer, 2001).

As mentioned before, research has shown that the treatment effects for the symptoms of medical and psychiatric disorders are attenuated for those patients with co-occuring personality pathology in contrast to those without. Studies have documented poorer treatment outcomes and health status, and higher rates of health care use and costs in patients with comorbid personality disorders (Gross et al., 2002; Moran et al., 2001; Rendu et al., 2002; van Asselt et al., 2007). In the clinical setting, the interaction with patients suffering from personality disorders can be very difficult. Clinicians often find themselves dealing with impulsivity, poor insight, frequent interruptions or dropout from treatment. The patients might also elicit strong emotional reactions in the clinicians, for example feeling overwhelmed or attacked. The fact that a lot of the behaviors and difficulties associated with a personality disorder is ego-syntonic, that is, that the patients often subjectively do not suffer from them or report on them, makes diagnosis and treatment more difficult. Hence, a lot of research has been conducted on assessment, theory and treatment of personality disorders. Specialized treatments have been developed (e.g. Bateman & Fonagy, 2004a; Clarkin, Yeomans & Kernberg, 1999; 2006; Linehan, 1993) and psychotherapy research has found improvement of these "difficult patients" in psychotherapeutic treatment (Bateman & Fonagy, 1999; Clarkin et al., 2001, 2007; Levy et al., 2006; Linehan et al., 1999).

A meta-analysis by Perry, Banon, and Ianni (1999) suggests that psychotherapy is an effective treatment for personality disorder and may be associated with up to a sevenfold faster rate of recovery in comparison with the natural history of disorders. Although treatment of personality disorders is unlikely to result in the development of a fully healthy personality structure, it is important to realize that clinically and socially meaningful change to personality structure and functioning can and does occur (Clarkin et al., 2007; Levy et al., 2006). When taking into account both the public health care costs, high level of treatment utilization (e.g. Skodol et al., 2005) of many of the patients with personality disorders, and also the subjective stress, psychosocial impairment and burden it places on those who suffer from them and around them, it is highly necessary to further develop diagnostic procedures and treatments for this patient group.

2 Kernberg's concept of personality organization

In the previous chapter, the category based assessment of personality disorders according to the Diagnostic and Statistical Manual of Mental Disorders (APA, 1994) was described and discussed. A possible alternative was proposed by conceptualizing personality pathology dimensionally, for example ranging from normal to abnormal personality. Kernberg emphasizes that it is necessary to combine both categorical as well as dimensional criteria in the classification of personality and personality pathology. He proposes that a psychoanalytic theory based both on structure and on symptoms constitutes a good base (Kernberg, 1998). Kernberg regards structural criteria essential in the diagnosis of personality pathology because present structural criteria are connected with a theory of psychic development. In this chapter, Kernberg's object-relations theory of personality will be summarized briefly, focusing on the key structural criteria. Then, his conceptualization of different levels of personality organization will be presented and related to the DSM personality disorders.

Kernberg's thinking has been influenced by several psychology schools from which he has incorporated concepts into his model. Among these are Freud's structural model (Freud, 1923), Jacobson's Ego psychology (1964; 1971) as well as Klein's (1940; 1945; 1946; 1957), Fairbain's (1952) and Mahler's object-relations theories (Mahler, 1968; Mahler, Pine & Bergman, 1975). In his approach, he has focused mainly on patients with severe personality disorders and character pathology.

Kernberg united the contributions from the different schools into one theory focusing on pathologies of internalized object relations. He has created a complex framework for understanding emotional development and psychological conflict and for locating psychopathology according to levels of severity (Kernberg, 1975; 1976; 1980; 1984; 2004). In Kernberg's theory, affects serve as the primary motivational system (Kernberg, 1982). For the development of personality pathology, he emphasizes the importance of early internalized object relations. He states that the internalization of dyadic units of self and object representations under the impact of peak affect states have significant implications for the psychoanalytic theory of drives, for the understanding of the etiology of identity diffusion and also for the psychoanalytic psychotherapy of severe personality disorders (Kernberg, 2005). Focusing on this theory of internalized object relations, a psychotherapeutic approach for the treatment of personality disorders located at borderline level (Clarkin, Yeomans, & Kernberg, 1999, 2006) as well as for the treatment of personality disorders at neurotic personality (Caligor, Kernberg & Clarkin, 2007) has been developed.

The Role of Internal Object Relations

In Kernberg's model, the organization of *psychological structures* depends on the interaction of constitutional and environmental factors early in life. A psychological structure is described as stable and enduring configuration of mental functions or processes that organize the individual's behavior and subjective experience. Pathological behaviors or symptoms shown by an individual therefore are hypothesized to reflect underlying disturbances of psychological structures (Kernberg & Caligor, 2005).

For the development of psychological structures, early *internalized object relations* play a key role. In patients with disturbances of psychological structures, one of the basic assumptions is that the patient's pathology is the unconscious repetition in the here-and-now of pathogenic internalized object relationships from the past. An internalized object relation is a self representation in relation to an object representation, linked through a particular affect. An example is the affect of love, linking the image of a childish-dependent figure with an ideal, giving figure. From the beginning of life, internal object relations are derived from the integration of inborn affect dispositions and interactions with caretakers.

Kernberg considers these *affect dispositions* as the primary motivational system. Affects are instinctive structures, psychophysiological in nature, biologically given and developmentally activated, which include psychic components. He proposes that affect dispositions are the bridging structures between biological instincts and psychic drives (Kernberg, 1992). Thus, in his theory, at the beginning there are no drives. Only through the course of time will good and bad experiences shape into the libidinal and aggressive drives Freud described. In Kernberg's theory, the child wants to maximize pleasurable experiences with good objects and destroy bad objects that provoke unpleasant experiences. He considers affects as the building blocks of drives; they eventually acquire a signal function for the activation of drives (Kernberg, 1984).

The centerpiece of his theory revolves around developmental levels of internal object relations, linked through affects. Almost immediately, affects are activated in relation to, regulated by and cognitively linked to interactions with caretakers. Over time, these early interactions between the child and his caretakers are internalized and gradually organized to form internal object relations. For example, if a child repeatedly experiences fear in the context of the interaction with the mother, an affective memory will be organized to form the enduring memory structure of a terrified self, linked by fear to a powerful mother. These internal object relations are regarded the basic building blocks of all mental experience.

In the early life of the infant, two series of internal object relations are developed, one series associated with highly charged positive affect states motivating "approach" behaviors, another associated with highly charged negative affect states motivating aversive behaviors. The core affect of aggressive internal object relations is rage. The dominant affects hatred and envy, which are seen in severe personality disorders, can be traced back to this core affect. In the pleasurable or sexual series of internal object relations, the core affect is primitive elation, gradually developing into sexual excitement and also evolving to organize dependency needs. During mental development, the opposite internal object relations are integrated and affect dispositions become better modulated. By joining the positive, libidinal affects and internal representation of the object, and the bad, aggressive affects and internal object representation, a more realistic image of the object may be obtained and may be integrated internally as whole object. Integration is facilitated by the development of cognitive capacities and ongoing learning regarding realistic aspects of the interaction between self and others under circumstances of low affect activation.

The integration of internal object relations is crucial for the development of psychological health. With individuals who fail at this developmental task, very intense, poorly integrated and poorly modulated forms of aggression as well as unintegrated representations of self and other will remain. These individuals are diagnosed at borderline level of personality organization. Only if contradicting internal object relations accompanied by the matching affect can be integrated, higher level structures can be developed and a more flexible affect modulation will follow. Different levels of pathology reflect the degree of integration of internal object relations.

These different levels are shown in the model of classification of personality pathology which Kernberg has developed. This model moves away from the categorical diagnosis of personality disorders and differentiates personality organization according to structural criteria (Kernberg, 1975;1984). Kernberg proposes a continuum of severity of pathology, moving from psychotic personality organization (PPO) to neurotic personality organization (NPO). In the middle one can find what he refers to as severe personality disorders or borderline personality organization (BPO). The main characteristics of the different levels of personality organization are summarized in table 2 (Kernberg, 1984). Following, the key structural criteria of Kernberg's model will be related to these different levels of personality organization.

Table 2. Differentiation of Personality Organization (from: Kernberg, 1984)

Structural Criteria	Neurotic	Borderline	Psychotic
Identity integration	Sharply delimited self and object representations. Integrated identity.	Identity diffusion. Contradictory aspects of self and others are poorly integrated and kept apart.	Self and object representations are poorly delimited.
Defensive Operations	Repression and higher level defenses: reaction formation, isolation, undoing, intellectualization. Defenses protect against intrapsychic conflict. Interpretation improves functioning.	Splitting and lower level defenses: Projective identification, idealization, omnipotence, denial, devaluation	Defenses protect from disintegration and self/object merging. Interpretation can lead to regression.
Reality Testing	Capacity exists to evaluate self and others realistically, in depth.	Alterations occur.	Capacity to test reality is lost.

Identity

The cornerstone of Kernberg's theory is the construct of identity. A normal, consolidated identity corresponds with the subjective experience of a stable and realistic sense of self and others and forms a fundamental precondition for normal self-esteem, self-enjoyment, the capacity to derive pleasure from work and values and an overall zest for life. Consolidated identity is associated with a broad array of affect dispositions and with the predominance of positive affect states. Parallel to the development of identity, another change in mental organization takes place; the formation of an integrated system of internalized values and morals, often referred to as "superego". The superego is seen as comprising successive layers of internalized self and object representations (Jacobson, 1964; Kernberg, 1984). The sequential integration of persecutory and idealizing representations, including the demands and prohibitions from the

parental figures in a realistic way, leads to the formation of a healthy superego and normal identity.
In contrast, pathological identity formation corresponds with an unstable, polarized and unrealistic sense of self and others. In this case, poorly modulated and intense, negative affects prevail. This development corresponds with the formation of a pathological superego. Very exaggerated ideals and positive values and an extremely persecutory quality of prohibitions can lead to splitting mechanisms at the level of internalized value systems and to antisocial behavior. In Kernberg's model, pathological identity is the result of failure in the task of integration of internal object relations and also leads to the corresponding disorganization of the system of internalized values.
Identity diffusion was described first by Erikson (1950; 1956) as essential in the diagnosis of personality pathology and developed further by many authors. Akhtar (1992) summarizes several clinical manifestations of identity diffusion; for example, contradictory character traits, the temporal discontinuity in the self, lack of authenticity, subtle body image disturbances, and feelings of emptiness. These aspects are strongly associated with a stable sense of self. Kernberg emphasizes that crucial elements of identity diffusion are not only the absence of a stable sense of self, but also the lack of internalized object representations (Kernberg, 1976). These unintegrated self and object representations are assessed in the Structural Interview (compare chapter II.3.2.) or the STIPO (compare chapter IV.2.1.), in order to elucidate the level of identity consolidation. For example, difficulties in the description of self and others as whole objects can demonstrate identity diffusion in a clinical interview. Moreover, in these interviews, the ability to invest in work and pleasure, the continuity across time and situations, as well as self esteem, are assessed as important indicators for identity consolidation versus pathology.
Consolidated identity is the hallmark of normal personality or higher level personality disorders ("neurotic personality organization"), whereas individuals with identity diffusion are located at borderline or psychotic personality organization. The level of identity integration is the most important differential criterion between neurotic personality organization and Borderline Personality Organization.

Defense Mechanisms

Another important dimension that differentiates between healthy or higher level, neurotic personality on the one hand, and borderline personality on the other is the use of predominant defensive operations. Individuals located at borderline or psychotic personality organization primarily use primitive defense mechanisms. The predominance of primitive defenses is associated with identity pathology and is developmentally connected to the stage of establishing specific affective memory structures, framed by the interaction between infant and caretaker. During this phase, structures associated with positive affects and affiliative behaviors are built up separately from those associated with negative affects and aversive behaviors. These positively and negatively charged affective experiences become dissociated from each other, leading to the separation of an idealized, "all good" sector and a persecutory, "all bad" sector. Failure to integrate idealized and persecutory mental structures leads to the use of "splitting" and related defensive operations. This serves to protect the idealized experiences from contamination with bad ones and to escape from the frightening experience of negative affect states (Kernberg & Caligor, 2005).

Primitive defense mechanisms are also predominant with patients located at psychotic personality organization, in which case use of the defenses protect the patient from further disintegration of the boundaries between self and object. Neurotic individuals primarily employ higher-level defenses based on repression, such as reaction formation, isolation or rationalization, all of which do not interfere with the integration of persecutory and idealized structures. These mechanisms protect the ego from intrapsychic conflicts rejecting a drive derivative or its ideational representation, or both, from the conscious ego. The emergence of defenses based on repression introduce a degree of rigidity into personality organization that is not seen in the normal personality (Kernberg & Caligor, 2005).

In interviews like the Structural Interview or the STIPO, the use of splitting and related defensive operations like primitive projection, projective identification, denial and omnipotent control is assessed in order to differentiate patients at borderline level from patients at neurotic level of personality. Also, the use of higher level defense mechanisms is examined by the STIPO, for example by exploring the ability for suppression or flexibility.

Reality Testing

Reality testing is defined as the capacity to differentiate self from nonself, intrapsychic from external origins of perceptions and stimuli, and the capacity to evaluate realistically one's own affect, behavior, and thought content in terms of ordinary social norms (Kernberg, 1984). Developmentally, the loss of reality testing reflects a failure of the separation of self image from object image, especially under conditions of peak affect activation. Individuals who fail at this first developmental task achieve no real boundary between their own mind and the experience and mind of others and are set up for a psychic fragmentation or a psychotic personality organization (PPO). In individuals with a neurotic personality structure (NPO), reality testing is preserved. With individuals at borderline level (BPO), reality testing is maintained and only somewhat reduced, shown primarily by a decreased capacity for subtle and tactful evaluation of interpersonal processes, especially in the setting of more intimate relations. Clinically, loss of reality testing is manifested in hallucinations and delusions. In interviews like the Structural Interview or STIPO, these phenomena are assessed by direct questions as well as through focusing on inappropriate affect or contradicting statements and on the patient's ability to empathize with others' thoughts, including the interviewer's perception of what the patient reported.

In sum, the most important differential criterion between patients located at psychotic personality organization and those presenting personality disorders is the level of impairment of reality testing. According to Kernberg's theory, with borderline patients, at times reality testing might be altered but never lost, as with psychotic patients. Next, what differentiates borderline organization from neurotic organization of personality is the level of identity consolidation and the defensive operations. Neurotic patients present with a healthier structure, they also show a more adaptive mode of affect regulation and higher level defenses. In contrast, patients with BPO present the syndrome of identity diffusion and have more immature ways of regulating their emotions, often presenting pathological aggression as well as utilizing primitive defense mechanisms. With regard to affective experiences, patients with severe personality disorders exhibit a limited array of affect dispositions and predominantly negative affect.

Therefore with these patients, the ability to form mature, non hostile relationships between self and others is lost or severely damaged.

Classification of personality disorders

The interrelation of Kernberg's classification of personality disorders and the DSM classification is shown in figure 1. Kernberg proposes a dimensional approach according to severity (Kernberg, 1976), moving from mild to extreme severity (shown vertically in the figure). The range of severity goes from psychotic personality organization through borderline personality organization to neurotic personality organization. Also, the dimension of introversion versus extraversion (shown horizontally) is important for the diagnostic process. Located across this matrix are the personality disorders which also are described in the DSM classification, as well as additional personality disorders which are not included in the DSM system.

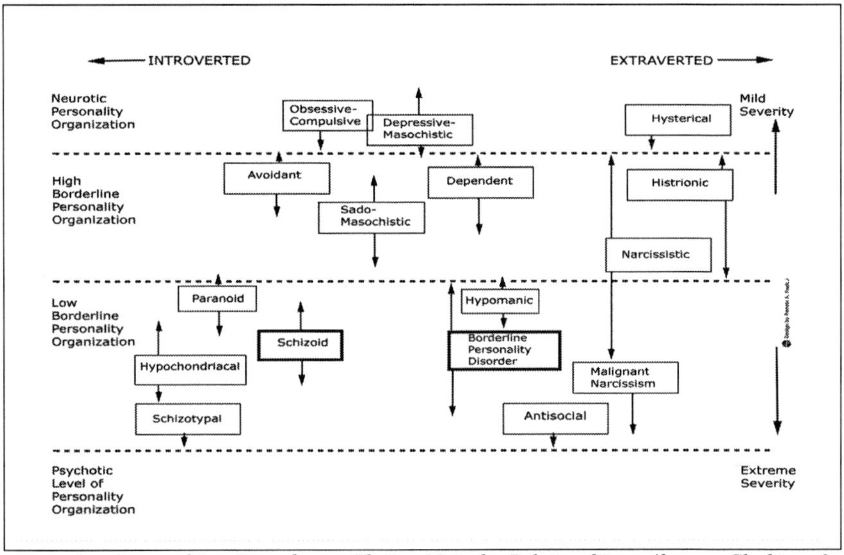

Figure 1. Personality Disorders: Their Mutual Relationships (from: Clarkin & Lenzenweger, 2005)

Differences from the DSM system. The first important difference between the two classification systems is Kernberg's use of the term personality organization; borderline personality *organization* is a much broader concept than just the borderline personality *disorder*. It comprises several personality disorders which share common features (i.e. identity diffusion, use of primitive defenses, maintained reality testing). Another difference to the DSM system (APA, 1994) is that Kernberg emphasizes the importance of several personality disorders which were not included in the DSM system. The most prominent one is the concept of malignant narcissism (Kernberg, 1992). An individual showing both antisocial and narcissistic features, accompanied by ego-syntonic aggression and paranoid traits, is diagnosed with the syndrome of malignant narcissism. Also, sadomasochistic personality disorder is an important disorder not included in the manual. Moreover, Kernberg also does not agree with the DSM system with regard to the diagnosis of avoidant personalities. Figure 1 includes this diagnosis in deference to DSM-IV, but Kernberg questions that the disorder exists as an diagnostic entity, because from his clinical experience he views them as variants of paranoid or schizoid personalities, expecting that all these personalities will change throughout time having more criteria in common with the other diagnoses (Kernberg, personal communication, May 2003).

Psychotic Personality Organization. According to Kernberg's model, all patients located at psychotic personality organization, characterized by identity diffusion and lack of reality testing, really represent atypical forms of psychosis. Strictly speaking, psychotic personality organization therefore represents an exclusion criterion when diagnosing personality disorders (Kernberg, 2000).

Personality Disorders at Borderline Personality Organization. In Kernberg's view, schizoid, schizotypal, paranoid, hypomanic, hypochondriacal, lower level narcissism, and antisocial personality disorders encompass the diagnosis of borderline personality disorder in the model of borderline organization. These personality disorders share certain features, centering on identity pathology, but are different on the dimension of extraversion – introversion. For example, in the schizoid personality, splitting mechanisms lead to deterioration of social relationships, apparent lack of affective experiences, and even to emptiness of the social life, exemplifying the introverted end of the spectrum. On the same level of severity, borderline personality disorders are at the extraverted end of the continuum. Individuals with borderline personality disorder act out their intrapsychic experiences in repetitive relationship patterns, often presenting lack of impulse control and affect storms (Kernberg, 2000).

Kernberg differentiates between lower level personality disorders and higher level BPO personality disorders. All these patients, located at BPO, suffer from identity diffusion, manifestations of primitive defenses and different degrees of super-ego degeneration. The most severe super-ego pathology is found in patients with antisocial personality disorder, lower level narcissistic personality disorder, and in patients with the syndrome of malignant narcissism. Although the whole group of BPO disorders shares the features of identity pathology and the use of primitive defenses and consequential difficulties in interpersonal relationships, a subgroup of patients is different: patients with higher level personality disorders, such as better functioning narcissistic, histrionic, or sadomasochistic personality disorders. These individuals are able to maintain a more satisfying form of social adaptation and usually are more successful in reaching a certain level of intimacy in object relations. Thus, these patients are located at a significantly less severe form of BPO.

Personality Disorders at Neurotic Personality Organization. Finally, Kernberg also describes higher level personality disorders, located (along with symptomatic neuroses; cf. Kernberg, 1984) at neurotic personality organization. These patients, for example individuals with obsessive-compulsive personality disorder, depressive-masochistic or hysterical personality disorder, present consolidated identity with the accompanying ability for deep object relations, more anxiety tolerance, and impulse control. As described previously, this group of patients does not employ primitive defenses but higher-level defenses.

In sum, Kernberg's model reflects how the process of diagnosing personality pathology should take place in two steps. First, personality pathology is conceptualized according to the dimension *severity of the pathology.* Then a second order diagnosis is made using a prototypic, or categorical, classification system, based on the key diagnostic structural criteria of each level of personality pathology. An important thought pertaining to the frequently found co-occurrence of personality disorders according to the DSM classification is that the underlying structural deficits shared by several types of personality disorders might well explain the overlap problem of symptoms of the different DSM diagnoses. Thus, the ordinary behavioral or phenomenological descriptions of patients can be supplemented by structural criteria which can sharpen the accuracy of the differential diagnosis of mental illness, especially in cases that are difficult to classify (Kernberg, 1984).

3 Diagnosis of personality disorders

After having presented personality disorders classified according to the Diagnostic and Statistical Manual of Mental Disorders and according to Kernberg's theory, now several instruments commonly used for the assessment of personality disorders will be presented. A variety of interview measures and self-reports exist, in this section the focus is set on assessments via interviews. Many researchers have commented on the fact that it is difficult to assess personality pathology, for example, due to socially desirable response patterns or poor insight on behalf of the patient. Often, interview measures are preferred to self-reports as they offer the opportunity to clarify questions, ask for examples of pathology or to verify that the pathology was not state specific but characteristic of long-term functioning. Also, the patient's behavior and demeanor can be observed during the interview as additional source of information (Zimmerman, 1994).
This list of diagnostic measures is clearly not exhaustive. Examples of interview measures will be discussed: first presenting the phenomenological approach of personality disorders through DSM-oriented methods, then describing the clinical interview Kernberg developed, and finally showing some interviews aiming at psychodynamically informed assessment or structural diagnosis. Besides these, other psychoanalytically oriented interviews were developed (cf. Mertens, 1992), for example the psychiatric interview by Sullivan (1954), the Tavistock interview by Balint and Balint (1961), the psychoanalytic initial interview (Argelander, 1970) or biographical anamnesis from a depth psychology perspective (Dührssen, 1981). To present all these methods is beyond the scope of this study; the described methods were chosen exemplarily and briefly will be compared.

3.1. Diagnostic assessment according to DSM classification

A problem in the diagnosis of personality disorders is that the reliability of clinically based personality disorder diagnoses is poor (e.g. Mellsop et al., 1982; Sartorius et al., 1993). For this reason, a number of structured or semi-structured interviews was created, enhancing the interrater diagnostic reliability of unstructured clinical evaluations. By including standardized questions concerning behaviorally-anchored diagnostic criteria in the interviews and using standardized rating and scoring, the diagnostic process could begin to provide a reliable outcome (Clarkin, 2003).

Skodol and colleagues (2002) report that semistructured clinical interviews have shown that interrater and test-retest reliabilities of BPD are substantially better than those obtained by clinical judgment alone (i.e., by unstructured clinical interviews). Examples for semistructured interviews are the *Diagnostic Interview for DSM-IV Personality Disorders (DIPD-IV)* (Zanarini et al., 1987; 2000), the *International Personality Disorder Examination (IPDE)* (Loranger et al., 1994; Loranger, Janca & Sartorius, 1997), the *Structured Interview for DSM-IV Personality (SIDP-IV)* (Pfohl, Blum & Zimmerman, 1997), the *Personality Disorder Interview – IV (PDI-IV)* (Widiger et al., 1995; Widiger & Frances, 1989), or the *Structured Clinical Interview for DSM-IV axis II Personality Disorders (SCID-II)* (First et al., 1995a; 1995b; 1996) It is currently unclear whether any of the interviews provides the most valid assessment and none is considered to be clearly superior to the others (Kaye & Shea, 2000).

These instruments assess the DSM-IV personality disorders based on criteria, analogous to the DSM-IV classification. Furthermore, the IPDE (Loranger, 1999; Loranger, Janca, & Sartorius, 1997) is an instrument compatible with the classification of personality disorders of both the DSM-IV and the ICD-10. It proved to be reliable and to show good temporal stability, and is applicable in samples across the world (Loranger et al., 1994).

In these structured interviews, separate for each personality disorder, a certain number of items has to be fulfilled to assign a diagnosis. For example, in the SCID-II, each item is rated on a 3-point scale with the values 1 (absent or false), 2 (subthreshold) to 3 (threshold), indicating the presence of personality disorder criteria. The amount of above-threshold fulfilled criteria determines if the diagnosis can be given. For example, to assign the diagnosis Borderline personality disorder, five out of nine criteria have to be fulfilled. An example for an item assessing Borderline Personality Disorder from the SCID-II is “Do you get into intense and stormy relationships with other people with lots of ups and downs?”, aiming at the DSM-IV criterion of “unstable and intense interpersonal relationships characterized by alternating between extremes of idealization and devaluation”.

The advantage of these structured, criterion-based assessments of personality disorders is the fact that they match psychiatric classification and are helpful for psychiatrists. Nevertheless, as mentioned above, the categorical approach (i.e. counting the amount of criteria for an assignment of a disorder) has been criticized for providing very heterogeneous concepts of the personality disorders, for not assessing levels of severity of the described disorders and also for being atheoretical. Furthermore, from a psychodynamic viewpoint, it is the assumption that pathological behaviors shown by patients may well represent very different functions or underlying structural deficits (Kernberg & Caligor, 2005). Thus, for many clinicians the unsatisfying classification according to DSM has caused them to develop other instruments, especially psycho-dynamically informed measures which also permit to use countertransference and following clinical cues for the diagnosis.

3.2. Kernberg's Structural Interview

One of the first interviews which is psychoanalytically informed and not geared to assess the diagnostic criteria of personality disorders according to DSM is Kernberg's *Structural Interview* (Kernberg, 1981, 1984). The development of several psychodynamic interviews stem from it and it has been applied by many clinicians (Buchheim et al., 1987). Kernberg developed this clinical interview to evaluate the aspects important to his psychoanalytic theory of personality organization, in particular to differentiate borderline personality organization from neurotic and from psychotic personality organization. Overall, the goal of this interview is the assessment of the following structural characteristics of the patient: consolidated identity versus identity diffusion, the relationship of primitive to advanced defenses, presence or absence of reality testing. In his Structural Interview, Kernberg connects the present functioning of the patient with the interaction of the patient with the interviewer.

The set-up of the interview follows a predetermined order (initial, middle and end phase), pursuing a circular order (compare the cycle of "anchoring symptoms" in Kernberg, 1984) which allows the interviewer, as he moves from one cardinal symptom to the next, to return eventually to the beginning and reinitiate a new cycle of inquiry. The specific questions and the order of questions are not predetermined, giving the interviewer flexibility to focus on relevant aspects and to return to important, perhaps contradicting issues.

In the initial phase, he covers the areas of symptoms and difficulties which brought the patient to the interview, and inquires about the expectations from the treatment and continues according to the reported symptoms. In this phase, the diagnosis of psychotic personality organization is tested. In the middle phase of the interview, the differential diagnosis of borderline versus neurotic personality organization is made. Crucial elements determining personality organization are evaluated: for example, identity consolidation versus identity diffusion are assessed by asking about self-description and description of others; important relationships provide the interviewer with information of the social situation and object relations. In this phase, the methods of clarification, confrontation and interpretation provide the interviewer with important prognostic and therapeutic information. At this point, the interviewer has to fulfill three tasks simultaneously: he must explore the internal world of the patient, at the same time observe the patient's interactions with the interviewer and also follow his own affective reactions and countertransference in order to understand the object relations activated by the patient. Throughout the interview, there is a focus on how the patient is functioning (i.e. thinking, assessing, processing questions, organizing answers) in the here and now interaction with the interviewer. For example, when aiming at determining the degree of impairment of reality testing, the interviewer might ask the patient about how he thinks that a particular aspect of his behavior is perceived by the interviewer. This clarification can yield meaningful information with regard to differential diagnosis: If a patient cannot discern that his behavior might seem odd to the interviewer, this can be seen as an indicator for impaired reality testing. In the final phase of the interview, Kernberg emphasizes leaving enough time to find out if any additional issues the patient considers important should still be discussed. Also, in this phase the necessity and the patient's motivation for further diagnostic or treatment steps can be evaluated and recommendations can be given.

Overall, the Structural Interview combines both psychoanalytic thinking and psychiatric exploration. The assessment both of clinical symptoms and of the level of personality organization provide the interviewer with important information for diagnosis, prognosis and further treatment planning.

3.3. Structured Interview of Personality Organization (STIPO)

As mentioned before, the reliability in unstructured clinical interviews is rather poor. While being a very sophisticated method and a clinically most useful tool, obtaining the same diagnostic results via Kernberg's Structural Interview can be difficult, especially for interviewers not so familiar with his theory. Thus, to increase diagnostic reliability, Clarkin, Caligor, Stern, and Kernberg have developed the *Structured Interview of Personality Organization (STIPO; 2004)* which is a semi-structured version of Kernberg's Structural Interview. It basically assesses the same domains as the Structural Interview, but provides clearly formulated questions and anchors aiding the scoring process and the classification of personality organization. The instrument assesses Kernberg's key domains which differentiate between levels of personality organization: identity, primitive defenses, reality testing, as well as other important dimensions (object relations, moral values, aggression). The design of the STIPO, including item samples and scoring procedures, will be explained in depth in section "IV. Methods", as it is the main instrument of this study. The validation process of the STIPO is still ongoing, part of which is this study, but first results suggest that it can reliably assess the constructs of personality pathology according to Kernberg's theory and that it can be used to make predictions helpful for the diagnosis of personality pathology and for treatment planning (Stern et al., 2004a; 2007; 2004b).

3.4. Karolinska Psychodynamic Profile (KAPP)

The *Karolinska Psychodynamic Profile (KAPP),* (Weinryb & Rossel, 1991) is an instrument based on psychoanalytic theory designed to assess relatively stable modes of mental functioning, as they appear in self-perception and in interpersonal relations. The information needed for assessment is obtained through a Structural Interview. The approach was developed from Kernberg's Structural Interview procedure (Kernberg, 1981; 1984).

The information obtained from the interview is rated on 18 scales. Quality of interpersonal relations is assessed by the subscales "intimacy and reciprocity", "dependency and separation", and "controlling personality traits". More specific aspects of personality functioning are captured in the subscales "frustration tolerance", "impulse control", "regression in the service of the ego" and "coping with aggressive affects". Two scales assess affect differentiation, both in experience and in expression, and three scales describe the importance attached to the body as a factor of self-esteem ("conception of bodily appearance", "conception of bodily functioning", "current body image"). The two subscales "sexual functioning" and "sexual satisfaction" explore sexuality, and the scales "sense of belonging", "feeling of being needed" and "access to advice and help" describe the individual's impression of his own social significance. Finally, on the last scale the individual's personality structure is described ("personality organization"). For each of the scales, a rating is done on a 3-point scale ranging from 1 ("most normal") to 3 ("least normal"), providing the additional possibility for intermediate levels on each scale.

The KAPP's construct validity was examined by comparing interview-based KAPP ratings with ratings based on projective measures and is reported as satisfactory, with correlations ranging from 0.33 to 0.82 (Weinryb, Rossel & Asberg, 1991a). Also, the ability of the KAPP to differentiate between patients with and without psychiatric disorder was confirmed (Weinryb et al., 1992). Interrater-reliability between interviewers at different levels of psychoanalytic training and familiarity with the instrument was examined by Weinryb and colleagues. The results indicate that the instrument has very high interrater-reliability, between 0.72 and 1.00 (Weinryb, Rossel & Asberg, 1991b; Weinryb et al., 1998). In sum, the KAPP demonstrated good reliability and validity. It has been translated into several languages and been influential in the development of other instruments, for example the OPD (Hoffmann, 1998).

3.5. Operationalized Psychodynamic Diagnostics (OPD)

Stemming from the need for a psychodynamic clinical classification that goes beyond the phenomenological and symptom oriented classification system of DSM-IV or ICD-10, the OPD task force developed the *Operationalized Psychodynamic Diagnostics (OPD)* (Arbeitskreis OPD, 1996; OPD Task Force, 2001). of which recently a second version has been published (Arbeitskreis OPD, 2006). The OPD is based on a multiaxial format, is theory-independent and is intended to promote communication within psychoanalysis and with related disciplines (Cierpka et al., 2007). OPD is thought to complement phenomenological classifications, focusing on implications for psychodynamic treatment planning and permitting both status and process diagnosis. The interview does not provide pre-determined questions, but should be held in a flexible manner, following five phases (Schauenburg, Janssen & Buchheim, 1998): the opening phase, followed by a phase focusing on experiences and episodes of interpersonal relationships, then moving on to the assessment of experience of self. In the fourth phase, the experience of others is examined and in the final phase, a summary and intervention can be given. During or after the interview, ratings are made on the five OPD axes, using anchor examples for each of the items. The OPD manual consists of five axes; four operationalized axes permitting the psychodynamic evaluation of a patient and one descriptive axis.

The first axis, "Experience of illness and prerequisites of treatment" focuses on the assessment of the experience of illness and the motivation for treatment, less on the descriptive behaviors and symptoms of illness. 20 items assess, among others, severity and duration of the somatic or mental illness, the degree the patient suffers from his symptoms, expectations from treatment, personal resources and psychosocial support, motivation for psychotherapy and for medical treatment, and secondary gain, are rated on a five-point scale (0 to 4). In the second version of the manual, for the measurement of severity, the General Assessment of Functioning Scale (GAF) from the DSM-IV (APA, 1994) and for the assessment of quality of life the EQ-5D (Rabin, de Charro2001) were added.

On axis II "Interpersonal relations", dysfunctional relationship patterns are assessed, based on narratives similarly to Luborsky's "Core Conflictual Relationship Theme Method (CCRT)" (Luborsky & Crits-Christoph, 1998). In part leaning on circumplex models like Benjamin's "Structural Analysis of Social Behaviors (SASB)" (Benjamin, 1974), this OPD axis is conceptualized as a circle, with two orthogonal and bipolar dimensions: interdependence (active: autonomy versus control, reactive: independence versus submissiveness) and affiliation (love versus hate). Interpersonal behaviors are described by 32 items (30 items in the first version of the manual; OPD-1) which are placed on an "active" and a "reactive" circle and are rated by the interviewer in formulations from four different perspectives: how the patient experiences his and others' behaviors in interactions as well as how others (including the interviewer) experience their interaction with him. By choosing up to three items for each of the four perspectives, a formulation of typical interpersonal interaction patterns for each patient can be made.

Axis III, "Conflicts", describes the degree of pervasive conflicts in different areas. The seven conflict themes are 1) "dependence versus autonomy", 2) "submission versus control", 3) "desire for care versus autarchy", 4) "self esteem conflicts", 5) "guilt conflicts", 6) "oedipal-sexual conflicts", 7) "identity conflicts", as well as the degree of the perception of conflicts and conflictual external stress, and are rated on a four-point scale (ranging from 0 "non-existent" to 3 "very important"). On this scale, changes from the first (1996) to the second manual (2006) include, among others, clearer operationalizations of the conflicts and the renaming of the first conflict into "dependence versus individuation".

On axis IV the psychic "structure" of the patient is assessed. On this axis, changes have been made from the first version (1996) to the second version (2006) of the OPD-system. In the first version, this axis consisted of six domains with subdomains and an overall rating. The dimensions were called 1) self-perception, 2) self-regulation, 3) defenses, 4) perception of others, 5) communication and 6) attachment. In the second version of the manual, modifications were made insofar as four scales and subscales were introduced, each with two directions (self- and other-directed). The major change was the abolishment of the domain defenses. In the current version of the manual, the four domains are 1) perception of self and others, 2) regulation of self and relationships, 3) internal and external communication, 4) attachment to internal and external objects. Each of these four domains consists of three subdomains, and anchor examples are given for each of the areas to be assessed. For each domain and subdomain, a rating is made based on the level of integration (ranging from (1) well integrated to (4) disintegrated) and a global rating of the structural level can be assigned.

Finally, axis V adds the description of mental and psychosomatic disorders according to ICD-10, assessing mental disorders as well as personality disorders and somatic disorders. This axis was included in deference to the common DSM-IV /ICD-10 classification system and is supposed to complement the psychodynamically oriented diagnoses on axis I to IV.

The reliability of the separate OPD axes was examined (Cierpka et al., 2007; Cierpka et al., 2001; Rudolf et al., 1996; Stasch et al., 2002) and good to satisfying scores for interrater agreement for the clinical context were determined, with reliabilities for the separate axes ranging from r=.30 to r=.50. The strongest values were found under routine conditions for the total evaluation of structure (.69) and for the selection of the two most important conflicts (.55). Significantly higher values were obtained when the OPD research interview served as the basis for the rating (weighted kappa: range .48-.81 for all axes), again the total evaluation of the structure demonstrated the best reliability (.70). Cierpka and colleagues (2001) concluded that the reliability of OPD for application in research was satisfactory for axes II and III and good for axis IV. The validity was examined in several studies (e.g. Cierpka et al., 2001; Mestel et al., 2004; Rudolf et al., 1996; Spitzer et al., 2002), and good results were found for each of the four axes for criterion, concurrent, predictive, construct and especially for clinical validity (see Cierpka et al., 2007 for an overview).

3.6. Comparison of the measures

When comparing these measures which all aim at assessing personality pathology, several questions will be considered. Where is the focus of assessment – symptoms or personality structure? Where are the differences between these instruments, both with regard to form and to content? What are the implications for treatment planning?

Form of assessment

Regarding the form of assessment, in a *DSM-based instrument* like the SCID-II, standardized questions are followed throughout the interview. The STIPO also uses standardized questions and provides a clearly structured order of domains and questions. Both in *KAPP* and *OPD*, the questions are partially predetermined, but largely follow the concept of a clinical Structural Interview. Although not based on pre-determined questions, the interviewer in the KAPP is instructed to pay attention that all aspects necessary for the evaluation of the 18 scales have been mentioned. The authors state that the *KAPP* is purposefully less specific and detailed in its scale descriptions and interview instructions than other psychoanalytic instruments, in order to allow interviewers who are well familiar with the KAPP but have less extensive training of the instrument to carry it out reliably (Weinryb, 1998). In the *OPD*, the interviewer should also keep in mind the different axes for which the information should be gathered and should follow the four phases of the OPD-interview (see above). Kernberg's *Structural Interview* is the least structured, not using predetermined questions; while the interviewer is provided with a sequence of domains to be assessed, he is still given a lot of flexibility to follow important leads of the individual patient.

This flexibility in the clinical interview is one of the main differences between the DSM-based instruments and the presented psychodynamically oriented ones: interviewers are asked to also follow their countertransference leads when determining what to assess next and how to rate or diagnose the patient. Countertransference is an important aspect in Kernberg's *Structural Interview*, in which the interviewer in large part is guided by his countertransference. Also the clinical *STIPO* ratings take into account both what the patient reports as well as the clinical impression. In the *KAPP*, clarifications and confrontations within the assessment, which are largely guided by countertransference impressions, are emphasized, similarly to the Structural Interview. In the *OPD*, especially on the axes "relational issues" (when rating how others, including the interviewer, experience the patient) and "structure", countertransference plays an important role. The final phase of the *OPD*, in which a summary and possibly an interpretation is given, shows similarities to the ending of the Structural Interview. *DSM- oriented measures* are more likely to take answers given by the patients at face value, whereas psychodynamically oriented instruments provide the interviewer with more freedom to weigh in his clinical impression or countertransference. This is an important aspect in the diagnostic process of patients with personality pathology, who often report contradicting or confusing information which can be complemented by the interviewer's clinical impression. In sum, the emphasis on countertransference and flexibility shown especially in the methods aiming at a structural diagnosis is an important vehicle of psychodynamic assessment; but these methods require a certain degree of clinical experience. The degree of interrater reliability is likely to be affected by this flexibility.

Content of assessment

What do the instruments have in common? First, it is obvious that the instruments based on the *DSM classification* (e.g. SCID-II) are quite different from the four other instruments presented. They focus on assessment of symptoms in order to assign a specific personality disorders diagnosis according to the classification of the DSM of ICD-system. Also in the *OPD*, on axis V, these syndromal diagnoses are given as well. The *Structural Interview, STIPO, KAPP* and the remaining axes of the *OPD* do not primarily focus on symptom assessment, although this, of course, is taken into consideration. For example, in the Structural Interview the interviewer asks for symptoms as part of the clinical evaluation. These instruments focus on the structural diagnosis, that is, exploring the level of personality organization beyond the behavioral manifestation of symptoms, from a psychodynamic point of view.

Furthermore, the *KAPP* and the *OPD* also have other foci of assessment. For example, the *OPD* explores the nature of dominant conflicts, which is not done by the *KAPP*, the *STIPO* or the *Structural Interview.* With regard to specific scales, strong overlap is suspected in the domains of axis IV of the *OPD* called "perception of self" and "perception of others" with the similarly named *STIPO* identity subdomains; the "defenses" scale of the *OPD* (which was part of axis IV only in OPD-1, but no longer in the second version OPD-2) might also correspond to the "primitive defenses" domain of the *STIPO*.

An interesting difference between these two instruments might be that in the *OPD* axis "structure" the focus is set on the best possible evaluation of the individual. This means that the "highest" level of structure, involving the level of highest functioning is assessed. A longer time frame is considered; for example, in order not to give too much weight to a phase of alcohol abuse in the previous year, but to aim at a more general assessment throughout the last years. Contrary to this, Kernberg's assessment in the *Structural Interview* or *STIPO* focuses on the lowest level. For example, by confronting the patient and by evaluating his ability to integrate conflicting aspects, the "most severe" degree of identity diffusion is assessed.

With regard to theoretical background, it is clear that the DSM is purposefully atheoretical in order to assess specific behaviors with a non-theoretical approach; whereas the *Structural Interview* follows Kernberg's theory of personality organization, and the *KAPP*, and especially the *OPD*, include a broad range of theoretical conceptualizations. The empirical overlap of these instruments remains to be explored. One of the main goals of this study is to examine the extent that the *STIPO* can operationalize Kernberg's theory.

The axis "structure" from the *OPD*, the results from Kernberg's *Structural Interview*, the final categorization from the *KAPP* as well as the level of personality organization obtained from the *STIPO* all seem to aim at similar contents. Future research could examine results obtained from these different instruments as they relate to each other, thus showing the degree of overlap and examining the concordant validity of the instruments.

Implications for treatment planning

An important goal of assessment is to issue a diagnosis or to provide implications for treatment. The authors of the DSM (American Psychiatric Association, 1994) admit that the diagnosis in and of itself does not provide a roadmap for treatment. Going beyond the mere assessment of behavioral symptoms and the diagnosis itself, the *Structural Interview*, the *STIPO*, the *OPD* and the *KAPP* do intend to assess other important information needed for treatment planning, especially the personality structure. Clarkin, Kernberg and Somavia (1998) propose to transform the results from an assessment based on a psychodynamic theory of personality and pathology into implications for treatment. This approach emphasizes the level of personality organization and the prominent object relations in addition to the assessment of behaviors and traits. For example, the level of aggression, the secondary gain and the degree of introspective abilities are important prognostic factors influencing the treatment planning. The structural level and corresponding degree of "analyzability" determines the choice of therapy, for example psychoanalytic psychotherapy versus psychoanalysis (Mertens, 1992). Both the *Structural Interview* and *STIPO* are based on Kernberg's underlying theory and take into consideration the implications for treatment. Also, the *OPD* puts a strong emphasis on therapy planning and derivatives from the assessment for treatment, for example assessing the prerequisites for treatment from the *OPD* axis I as a guideline for treatment. Further on, it seems helpful to use the information obtained during the interview regarding the dominant relationship patterns (axis II) to conclude what this could mean for the therapeutic relationship. Another important step in treatment planning, in the assessment of psychic structure and measurement of change was done by members of the OPD task force. Based on the OPD, a model has been developed in which individual problem areas for each patient may be chosen from a list of foci, and changes in these foci are evaluated using a scale called the *Heidelberg Structural Change Scale* (Grande et al., 2001; Rudolf, Oberbracht & Grande, 1998).

In sum, the structural level with corresponding foci of deficits and resources, assessed for example in the *Structural Interview*, the *OPD* axis IV or scale 18 of the *KAPP*, can be seen as an important differential marker for treatment planning. This study is part of an ongoing examination on the validity of the STIPO, which also will relate to treatment planning. The ability of the STIPO and the prototype derived from it for differential treatment planning will be investigated exemplarily in section V.2., the single case analysis.

4 The prototype concept

After presenting several conceptualizations of personality disorder and the corresponding methods of diagnosing them, the key question of this study is addressed: based on Kernberg's model of different levels of personality organization, would a prototype model of BPO be helpful in the diagnosis of BPO? For this reason, several other prototype approaches will be summarized and will be related to the objective of this study, the development of a prototype of BPO.

Classical versus prototype categorization

In certain respects, the concept of diagnosing personality disorders as done with the DSM system (American Psychiatric Association, 1994) is a prototype method. For example, in order to obtain the diagnosis BPD, a patient must fulfill 5 out of 9 prototypic diagnostic criteria. The description of the criteria for the diagnosis BPD therefore is considered a prototype; a patient will more or less match this prototype. Cantor et al. (1980) describe how with DSM-III diagnoses, psychiatric classification moved toward *prototype categorization*, away from *classical categorization*. The classical system of categorization defines category membership being determined by a small set of singly necessary and jointly sufficient features and anything that has these features being a member of the category. For example, in the case of the abstract category "square", all squares have four equal sides joined at right angles. Thus, the classical view assumes distinct boundaries and homogenous membership within one category, whereas in a prototype view larger sets of correlated features constitute the classification. Prototypes make sense out of variations in typicality and therefore result in heterogeneity of the symptoms of like-diagnosed patients and in absence of

distinct boundaries. Cantor and colleagues state the importance of a prototype view as this way the probabilistic nature of diagnostic categorization is emphasized. They deduce that "utilization of confidence/typicality ratings in diagnosis can be encouraged and diagnoses can be made on the basis of degree of fit between the patient's cluster of symptoms and the prototypes for various different categories" (Cantor et al., 1980, p.192). Also, treatment programs could be designed to match the degree of typicality of the patient. Cantor and colleagues found in an investigation with experienced clinicians that prototypes associated with basic-level diagnostic categories (e.g. schizophrenia versus affective disorder) were more distinctive than prototypes for the less inclusive lower level categories. This thought of using broader, more inclusive basic level diagnostic categories rather than distinguishing between patients that fit in more than one of the substantially overlapping lower level categories is closely related to the concept of the prototype of BPO developed in this study.
Regarding the diagnosis of Borderline Personality Disorder according to DSM, the prototype approach was empirically examined by Clarkin and colleagues (1983). They conclude that the diagnosis of BPD is consistent with a prototypical model of classification, shown by heterogeneous membership within the category and by absence of distinct boundaries with many borderline cases and overlapping diagnoses. Conditional probabilities showed the differential efficiency of the single diagnostic criteria of BPD. Some criteria predicted the diagnosis BPD better than others, especially the criteria "unstable/intense relationships" and "identity disturbance". The results indicate the importance of assessing the conditional probabilities both of individual symptoms and of the combination of symptoms. Also, one might conclude that due to the differential diagnostic value of the diagnostic criteria, a broader concept of underlying pathology could be useful for the diagnosis of personality pathology.

SWAP prototypes of personality disorders

Apart from these considerations examining classical versus prototypical models, efforts were made to establish clinical prototypes in order to make diagnosis of personality pathology easier. Two approaches will be illustrated more in detail as they show similarities to the approach used in this study. Westen and Shedler (2000) described a prototype matching approach to diagnosis based on a psychodynamic instrument, the *Shedler-Westen Assessment Procedure (SWAP).*

The SWAP is a Q-sort instrument that allows clinicians to describe a patient's personality organization based on two hundred statements that the clinician arranges into categories according to their relevance (Westen & Shedler, 1999a; Westen & Shedler, 1999b). A taxonomy of personality disorders was developed by asking a large number of clinicians to use the SWAP-200 to describe either actual patients or hypothetical, prototypical patients with one of the DSM personality disorders. By means of Q-factor-analyses, the data yielded aggregated descriptions of actual patients in each diagnostic category as well as aggregated descriptions of hypothetical, prototypical patients. Based on the descriptions of actual patients (Westen & Shedler, 1999b), seven Q-factors were defined representing independent naturally occurring categories of personality pathology some of which show similarities to the DSM personality disorders, while others go beyond the DSM categories (e.g. antisocial Q-factor, paranoid Q-factor, histrionic Q-factor, dysphoric Q-factor). In a next step, five additional subcategories of the dysphoric category were established through a second Q-analysis. In addition, by averaging or compositing hypothetical, prototypical patients, 15 diagnostic prototypes were created; one for each of the 14 DSM personality disorders (10 disorders currently in axis II, also four disorders in the appendix or in the previous version of DSM) and one for healthy, high functioning patients (Westen & Shedler, 1999a).

The SWAP can be used in two ways. First, an individualized personality portrait can be obtained by arranging the statements into eight categories, from those that are not descriptive (assigned a value of "0") to those that are highly descriptive (assigned a value of "7") and focusing on the statements that receive the highest rankings. Second, the degree of similarity of the individual patient to each of empirically derived prototypes (Westen & Shedler, 1999a) can be measured. This can be done mathematically by computing the correlation coefficient, called a personality disorder score. For each patient, 15 dimensional personality disorder scores can be computed, one for each diagnostic prototype. The personality disorder scores indicate how closely a patient matches the diagnostic prototype for each personality disorder. Westen and Shedler (2000) state that computing the correlation of SWAP-200 descriptions with personality disorder scores in order to assess the similarity to the prototype might be too cumbersome for day-to-day clinical practice but useful for research purposes. They conclude that for clinical purposes, the empirically derived Q-factors serve as diagnostic templates against which a given patient's SWAP-200 description is compared to assess degree of match (ranging on a scale from (1) no match to (5) very strong match). Also, a threshold for the categorical assignment of a diagnosis can be chosen. This way, both dimensional and categorical assessments (above-threshold vs. below-threshold) can be made. They suggest using this template-matching approach alternatively to the DSM symptom counting approach in clinical practice. In a recent study, Westen and colleagues (Westen, Shedler & Bradley, 2006) report that their prototype matching approach reduced findings of comorbidity relative to DSM-IV diagnosis without decrements in validity and outperformed DSM-IV diagnosis in ratings of clinical utility and ease of use.

FFM prototypes of personality disorders

Prototypes of personality disorders based on the FFM have been studied by proponents of the Five-Factor-Model of Personality (FFM) to demonstrate the clinical usefulness of the FFM. Lynam and Widiger (2001) asked researchers to rate a prototypic case of the respective DSM personality disorders in the language of the FFM. This method yielded an expert consensus profile for each of the 10 DSM-IV personality disorders. The researchers provided descriptions of personality disorders that they had studied by using descriptions from the domains and facets of the FFM. For example, antisocial personality disorder was represented by low scores on all 6 facets of agreeableness, 3 of 6 facets of conscientiousness (dutifulness, self-discipline, deliberation) and 2 facets of neuroticism (anxiousness and self-consciousness). It also was represented by high scores on 3 of the 6 facets of extraversion and 2 facets of neuroticism (angry hostility and impulsiveness). High interrater reliability and close agreement between the researchers' profiles and the FFM profiles of DSM personality disorders as described by Widiger et al. (1994) were reported.

While Lynam and Widiger (2001) examined prototypes of personality disorders based on the consensus of a large group of researchers, Samuel and Widiger (2004) inspected prototypes of personality disorders based on the consensus of practicing clinicians with personal experience in treating each respective personality disorder. They conclude that the consensus ratings on personality disorders both from researchers and from clinicians show that personality disorders can be conceptualized according to the FFM model. As mentioned before, the applicability of the FFM to clinical practice has been questioned by some authors (e.g. Benjamin, 1993).

The aforementioned studies examined the whole array of DSM personality disorders. Others have focused on individual personality disorders; for example Miller and colleagues (Miller et al., 2001) assessed psychopathy by the degree of similarity between an individual's results in the self-report measure *Revised NEO Personality Inventory (NEO-PI-R)* (Costa & McCrae, 1992b) and an expert-generated FFM psychopathy prototype. Their results indicate that psychopathy can be understood as an extreme variant of common dimensions of personality. Finally, Trull and colleagues (2003) specifically examined a prototype of BPD: they matched the FFM prototype of BPD reported by Lynam and Widiger (2001) to individuals' results on the NEO-PI-R to yield a "similarity score". This similarity index was then compared empirically with existing measures of BPD across a variety of samples and hypothesized correlates like measures of dysfunction or history of childhood abuse. The FFM BPD index correlated as high with these measures as they did with one another, emphasizing the validity of a valid FFM index.

A prototype of BPO

Our study's methodology leans on the methodology of the study by Trull et al. (2003) to a certain degree. Also, an expert consensus is developed, but instead of focusing on BPD, in this study, Kernberg's concept of Borderline Personality Organization (BPO) will be tested. Similarly to the FFM profile of BPD, in our study a profile of BPO based on the clinical scales of the STIPO is examined empirically. The closeness of each patient to this profile results in a STIPO-based BPO similarity index. At this step, a comparable process to Westen and Shedler's prototype development (Westen & Shedler, 1999a; Westen & Shedler, 2000) also can be seen: they examined the degree of similarity of each patient to several empirically derived prototypes. They obtained a correlation coefficient for each personality disorder, which in a way could be considered comparable to the BPO similarity index of this study. An important difference to the FFM approach and also the SWAP approach is that our similarity index is based on a *theoretically based concept* of BPO, aiming at the assessment of personality structure. In contrast, both FFM and SWAP develop their prototypes empirically, the FFM prototypes are lexically derived and the SWAP prototypes include a broad range of descriptions which are also theoretically informed but primarily clinically-oriented. Also, we examine a prototype of a broader concept, namely a level of personality organization, which cuts across most of the DSM personality disorders. Both the FFM and the SWAP prototypes are specific to the respective DSM personality disorders.

In sum, the goal of this study is to examine a prototype, specifically of BPO, and test its usefulness in focusing on the most relevant aspects of personality organization. The BPO prototype developed in this study based on Kernberg's conceptualization of BPO (1981) hypothesizes that all BPO patients share specific features to a certain degree, i.e. impaired identity, use of primitive defenses, overall stable reality testing. The degree of common pathology in these features is examined by comparing the patients to a prototypical profile of BPO; a *prototype of BPO.* Of course, the phenomenological characteristics of patients with BPO are expected to vary, in line with Kernberg's thinking (1975). Also, the degree of impairment in these domains is likely to differ within the population of BPO patients, and we are interested in examining variation of levels of pathology. Furthermore, we expect this BPO-prototypical pathology to differentiate this group of patients from another group (i.e. Neurotic Personality Organization).

The diagnosis of personality pathology and differential treatment planning could be aided by identifying a patient's closeness to a theoretically derived BPO prototype. It may help in identifying the crucial strengths and deficits a patient presents and assist in developing a guideline for treatment. With regard to the development of the STIPO, it is likely to shorten the interview to a screening instrument and help focus on the most relevant aspects of personality organization.

III GOALS AND HYPOTHESES

1 <u>Goals</u>

The general goal of this study is to test a prototype of Borderline Personality Organization (BPO) derived from the clinical scales of the *Structured Interview of Personality Organization (STIPO; Clarkin et al., 2004)* and thus, to examine the utility of the STIPO in explaining variance in personality disorders symptoms and correlates (e.g., negative affect, aggression). Confirmation of the hypotheses discussed below would suggest that the STIPO and the prototype derived from this instrument could be useful in the assessment and treatment of patients with personality disorders, and be a useful tool for the scientific study of personality pathology.

The specific goals of this study are

1) to develop a BPO prototype based on an expert-consensus. This BPO prototype should discriminate between patients located at the level of borderline personality organization and patients belonging to the neurotic personality organization.
2) to construct a BPO similarity index reflecting the differences between individual STIPO scores on the included variables, and prototype scores on those same variables.
3) to examine the BPO prototype's utility in discriminating between different patient groups, showing different levels of pathology on external variables of general functioning, axis I symptoms and axis II symptoms and correlates.
4) to test the interrater reliability of the clinical ratings of the BPO prototypical domains.
5) to establish the convergent validity of the BPO index by correlating the similarity index from each patient of a clinical sample with other measures of personality disorder and with correlates of personality disorder (for example, negative affect or aggression) and by correlating the similarity index from each patient with measures of positive affect and temperament.
6) to test the incremental validity of the BPO index by comparing the ability of the BPO similarity index to predict axis II symptomatology over and above two different measures relevant to axis II. In the first regression model testing the incremental validity of the BPO similarity index, a measure of the FFM, the *Big Five Inventory-44* (BFI-44; John, Donahue & Kentle, 1991) is first entered into the regression model. In the second test, the self-report

instrument *Inventory of Personality Organization* (IPO; Clarkin, Foelsch & Kernberg, 2001) is entered prior to the similarity index. These tests determine whether unique variance in BPO symptoms and correlates is explained by the STIPO-derived BPO similarity index above the BFI-44 and the IPO, and, in the second test, whether the interview method explains additional variance over and above a questionnaire tapping content similar to the STIPO. Demonstration of incremental validity over the BFI-44 would suggest the STIPO's utility in diagnosing personality pathology in addition to a model, the five-factor model of personality, whose relation to axis II is well-documented. Demonstration of incremental validity over and above the IPO, a self-report measure assessing content similar to the STIPO, would demonstrate construct validity and show that additional variance can be explained by the interview method alone.

2 Hypotheses

As mentioned in the previous section, after establishing the BPO similarity index based on the BPO prototype, its validity should be tested. The decision was made to examine the convergent and incremental validity of the BPO index. The discriminant validity concerning other personality disorders will not be considered. This was done by Trull and colleagues (2003) who established the discriminant validity of their FFM index of BPD as it correlates with the individual personality disorders avoidant personality disorder or antisocial personality disorder. Due to the concept of a broad-spectrum Borderline Personality Organization (BPO), which comprises most of the personality disorders as listed in the fourth edition of the Diagnostic and Statistical Manual of Mental Disorders (DSM-IV; APA, 1994), and the assumption that they share common structural features, we would not expect to differentiate the individual personality disorders within BPO, and aiming at discriminant validity, we do not expect strong differences when examining the correlation between the BPO similarity index and the individual personality disorders.

2.1. Hypothesis 1: Differentiation between clinical groups through BPO prototype

The BPO prototype is expected to discriminate between relevant clinical groups in a sample of patients, according to levels of pathology assessed with "General Assessment of Functioning" (GAF) and BSI Scale "General Severity Index", levels of axis I pathology assessed with the BSI subscales, and levels of axis II pathology measured with IPO, SNAP and other relevant external measures.

2.2. Hypothesis 2: Interrater reliability of the BPO prototype

We hypothesize high interrater-reliability for the clinical ratings of the STIPO domains which the BPO prototypical profile consists of.

2.3. Hypothesis 3: Convergent validity of the BPO similarity index

The BPO Similarity Index is expected to show a high correlation with measures of axis II pathology (i.e. SNAP Scales), and also with correlates of axis II (e.g., IIP-PD, negative temperament and aggression). The BPO Similarity index also should have an inverse correlation with measures of positive temperament and affect (e.g. SNAP Positive Temperament, BFI agreeableness, PANAS positive affect).

2.4. Hypothesis 4: Incremental validity of the BPO similarity index

We anticipate that the BPO Similarity Index will account for significant portions of variance in axis II symptoms and correlates. We also hypothesize, based on the findings of Trull et al. (2003), that the variables of the *Big-Five-Inventory-44* (BFI-44; John, Donahue, & Kentle, 1991), an instrument of the Five-Factor-Model of Personality, as a group will as well explain significant portions of the variance in axis II symptoms and correlates. In testing the incremental validity of the BPO similarity index, we hope to find that the index explains unique, additional portions of the variance in relevant variables after accounting for variance explained by the BFI-44.

2.5. Hypothesis 5: Incremental validity of the BPO similarity index

We anticipate that the BPO Similarity Index, which is derived from the interview measure STIPO, will account for significant portions of variance in axis II symptoms and correlates. The *Inventory of Personality Organization* (IPO; Clarkin, Foelsch, & Kernberg, 2001) is the self-report precursor of the STIPO and we expect the interview measure assessing personality organization to allow for a more in-depth, clinical assessment than the self-report, and expect the quality of the data to have greater accuracy. Thus, we hypothesize that the STIPO will explain additional variance over and above the IPO. In testing the incremental validity of the BPO similarity index, we hope to find that the index explains unique, additional portions of the variance in validity variables after accounting for variance explained by the IPO.

IV METHODS

1 Subjects and Procedures

The subjects were patients in inpatient, outpatient or private practice treatment who were recruited as part of an ongoing study concerning the instrument development of the STIPO (Stern et al., 2007). Before the empirical part of the study started, the theory-based expert consensus on BPO was formed which was then to be evaluated empirically through the different modes of assessment. For this purpose, I had regular meetings with the experts on BPO, Dr. Kernberg and Dr. Caligor, who found an agreement on the prototypical profile. Then, the empirical part of the study began. Before conducting the STIPO interviews and testing, I underwent an extensive training in the STIPO Interview and rating procedures. I was taught by the authors of the instrument and by experienced interviewers of the Personality Disorders Institute by going through an elaborate reliability training: The training consisted of teachings about the content and background of the instrument as well as watching video-taped interviews done by the authors and also attending interviews they did with patients at the Personality Disorders Institute: We rated all of these interviews individually, then we compared the ratings and discussed the results. In the next step, I received personalized feedback after conducting my own interviews which were videotaped and discussed with the authors of the interview. Also, I obtained training in evaluating and interpreting the self-report measures (e.g. SNAP, IIP-PD, Buss-Durkee Inventory) the patients were to fill out as part of the study.

The subjects were recruited between April 2003 and May 2004 on the units and Out Patient Department of the New York Presbyterian Hospital (NYPH) of Cornell University or referred to by clinicians associated with the Personality Disorders Institute of Weill Medical College of Cornell University. During the assessment period, I regularly contacted patients on the inpatient units or the Outpatient Department of the hospital, as well as got in touch with the patients referred to from the private practices. Two appointments with each of them were scheduled, one for the STIPO interview, one for the filling out of the self-report forms. The patients were informed that the interview would be videotaped and that they would be paid $25 for the testing. The patients were screened for the inclusion criteria, which were age of 18 and older and having no active DSM-IV bipolar disorder or psychotic disorder. After accepting the study conditions by signing an informed consent, they spent approximately two hours for the interview and two hours for filling out the questionnaires. The interviews were conducted in rooms of the units of the hospital or in the Personality Disorders Institute. Feedback concerning each patient's results from the testing was passed to the respective therapist on the patient's request.

2 Measures

Demographic data (age, educational level, gender, employment status, relationship status) was assessed by a demographic questionnaire. Ratings on the General Assessment of Functioning scale (GAF, from the DSM-IV, APA, 1994) were assigned for each patient by clinicians independent from the interviewers. Furthermore, history of previous hospitalizations, history of self-injurious behavior and history of suicide attempts was assessed by chart review in a binary format (yes-no). In addition to this data, the following interview and self-report measures were administered.

2.1. Structured Interview of Personality Organization

The *Structured Interview of Personality Organization* by Clarkin, Caligor, Stern, and Kernberg (2004) is a semi-structured interview developed to evaluate the individual's personality organization according to the psychodynamic conceptualization of Kernberg (1996). It permits the clinician to make a categorical and a dimensional assessment. First, subjects can be described as falling within the normal, neurotic or borderline range of personality organization. Second, the personality organization is assessed in seven domains. The interview examines the areas of identity consolidation, quality of object relations, use of advanced or primitive defenses, nature of reality testing and perceptual distortions, quality of aggression and moral values. The STIPO examines both the individual's internal world and behavioral world by inquiring about behaviors (for example the behavior with coworkers at work) and subjective experiences (e.g. perception of others) and aims at complementing both perspectives.

2.1.1 ***Background***

As described in chapter II. 3., several efforts have been made to diagnose personality disorders and personality structure. The direct precursor to the STIPO was Kernberg's *Structural Interview* (Clarkin, Kernberg & Somavia, 1998; Kernberg, 1981) which is a basically unstructured interview in which the interviewer mainly relies on his clinical knowledge and experience. The STIPO was developed in order to give clinicians more guidance when assessing psychic structure and structural change. *The Inventory of Personality Organization* (IPO) was a step in the development of the STIPO as it is a self-report instrument operationalizing Kernberg's theory of personality organization and examining similar domains. One of the research questions of this study investigates the overlap between the IPO and the STIPO by testing a STIPO-derived prototype of BPO.

2.1.2 ***Categorical assessment – Personality Structure***

The structural diagnosis is one of the major goals of the STIPO. The categorical assessment of personality organization is based on the key ego functions identity formation, defenses and reality testing. Patients who fall into the normal and neurotic range have a consolidated identity, intact reality testing, and use higher level defenses. Patients in the borderline range do not have a consolidated identity ("identity diffusion"), use primitive defenses and have variable reality testing. Fixed impairment in reality testing distinguishes patients presenting with atypical psychosis from those falling in the borderline range. Like the borderline group, patients with atypical psychosis present with identity diffusion. The decision at which level of personality organization the subject should be located is aided by the ratings made during the interview in the dimensional clinical ratings of these key domains.

2.1.3 ***Dimensional assessment – Domains of Personality Structure***

The seven dimensions of the STIPO will be described now, listing both the domains and the subdomains of the interview. Examples of answers to the individual items and the corresponding scoring can be found in section V.2. with each of the single cases. The STIPO score form is shown in the appendix. The seven domains are graphed in a profile of personality organization (figure 2) at the end of this section, horizontally showing the areas of assessment and vertically, the location on the dimensional scale of pathology (1= absence of pathology to 5= very severe pathology).

Identity

Identity is a descriptor of both the organization and the contents of the subject's inner world. An integrated and stable inner experience of self and others is responsible for the subjective sense of a cohesive self and also corresponds to the construct of identity, along with its behavioral correlates such as a capacity for investment in work and in stable, intimate relationships. Similarly, an unintegrated and unstable experience of self and others is responsible for the subjective sense of not having a cohesive self and also corresponds to the construct of identity diffusion, along with its behavioral correlates. Thus, a consolidated identity corresponds to an inner world in which experiences of self and others are well integrated and have depth and subtlety, that is, have the qualities of "whole objects" and are relatively stable over time. Identity diffusion corresponds to an inner world in which experiences of the self and others are polarized, contradictory and superficial, that is, have the quality of "part objects" and are unstable.

Identity is assessed in the STIPO by examination of the individual's investments in work or studies and free time activities (subdomain "Investments"), the degree of integration and stability of sense of self (subdomain "Coherent sense of self") and the nature of self-esteem regulation (subdomain "Self-valuation"). Identity is also assessed by examination of the subject's sense of others, the degree of integration and stability in the experience of others, along with the capacity to evaluate others in depth, beyond their transitory, experienced behaviors, and to accurately perceive what others are feeling and thinking (subdomain "Representation of others"). The presence of a poorly consolidated identity distinguishes the borderline level of organization from the neurotic level of organization.

Examples for questions assessing Identity are:

- *"How would you describe yourself to me so that I get a live and full picture of the kind of person you are?"* (Self-description)
- *"Would you say that your sense of who you are, or of what kind of person you are changes across different situations or time, for example, does it change according to where you are or who you're with?"* (Self-consistency across time)

- *"Is it hard for you to figure out what people think about you, what qualities in you they appreciate or dislike, or how they view you?"* (Other's judgments)

Object relations

Quality of object relations refers both to the quality of the subject's interpersonal relationships and to the nature of the subject's inner experience of self and others in interaction. Intrapsychically, quality of object relations is described in terms of the stability, degree of integration and depth of the subject's inner experience of self and others in interaction and in terms of the capacity for investment in relationships. Quality of object relations is assessed in the STIPO by examining the nature and stability of interpersonal (subdomain "Interpersonal relationships") and intimate relations, the ability to combine tenderness with erotism (subdomain "Intimate relationships/ Sexuality"), the subject's tendency to view relationships in terms of need fulfillment, ability for empathy and capacity to maintain a commitment to others over time (Subdomain "Internal working models of relationships").
Examples for questions assessing Object Relations are:

- *"Do you have relationships with friends consistently, over an extended period of time?"(*Interpersonal relationships- temporal stability)
- *"Do you find it difficult to experience tender feelings while still enjoying sex?"* (Sexuality- Love and Sex)
- *"Do you find it difficult to be supportive, or to comfort friends or family members who are in emotional pain?"* (Empathy)

Primitive Defenses

Defenses are the habitual reactions that the subject uses to ward off anxiety. The STIPO assesses the use of both advanced and primitive defenses. Primitive defenses, such as splitting, idealization/devaluation, primitive denial, projective identification, somatization and fantasy are characteristic of individuals with borderline personality organization. The STIPO assesses primitive defenses by inquiring about the conscious, subjective affective, cognitive and behavioral correlates of the use of primitive defensive operations.
Examples for questions assessing Primitive Defenses are:

- *"Are you someone who is cautious about other people, or who is often concerned about people's motives?* " (Paranoia)

- *"Are people regularly surprised by your behavior?"*(Erratic behavior)
- *"Do you find that your feelings for people tend to shift rapidly, for example, with you seeing them at times as one kind of person, and other times as a very different kind of person?"* (Idealization- Devaluation)

Coping and Rigidity

Advanced defenses, such as suppression and anticipation, and neurotic defenses, such as repression, intellectualization, reaction formation and displacement, are the predominant defenses used by individuals in the normal-neurotic range. Normals rely predominantly on advanced defenses, which are both flexible and adaptive. Neurotics rely predominantly on neurotic defenses, which are rigid, often cause psychological distress, and are less adaptive than advanced defenses. Coping refers to the individual's capacity to flexibly and adaptively respond to situations that are potentially stressful. An adaptive response, reflecting successful coping, will minimize psychological distress while responding appropriately and constructively to external circumstances. Rigidity refers to the chronic tendency to respond to potentially stressful situations in an automatic and stereotyped way that is to some degree maladaptive. A maladaptive response, reflecting character rigidity, causes psychological distress and does not necessarily lead to an optimal response to external circumstances. The STIPO assesses coping and rigidity by assessing how the individual anticipates and responds to stressful, challenging and disappointing situations, as well as the degree to which the individual is able to tolerate being in situations that are outside of his control.
Examples for questions assessing Coping and Rigidity are:

- *"When you make a mistake or something goes wrong, are you the kind of person who tends to blame yourself for it?"* (Self Blame)
- *"Are you the kind of person who needs to do things in a particular way, or who has a need to have things done "my way"?* (Control)

Aggression

Quality of aggression refers to the extent to which the subject's inner life and external behavior are dominated by aggression and defenses against aggression. Aggression is assessed in the STIPO by examining self-destructive and suicidal behavior (Subdomain "Self-directed aggression"), as well as sadism, omnipotent control of others and hatred (subdomain "other-directed aggression").

Examples for questions assessing Aggression are:

- *"Do you hurt, cut or cause physical pain to yourself? Do you get relief from tension by hurting yourself?"* (Relief)
- *"Do you lose your temper with others?"* (Temper)
- *"Do you find that you use hurting yourself, or threatening to hurt yourself, to get what you want from others, or to control others?"* (Threat of self injury)

Moral Values

Moral values refers to the extent to which the subject has internalized stable values and morals that affect his inner experience and guide his behavior. Morality and values are assessed in the STIPO by examining the subject's behavior in relation to moral decision-making and the capacity for guilt.

Examples for questions assessing Moral Values are:

- *"Are you confused about what to do when it comes to things like lying, stealing, or cheating if you think you can get away with it?"* (Internalized moral values)
- *"When you do something that goes against your sense of what is right, do you feel badly?"* (Guilt)

Reality Testing and Perceptual Distortions

Reality testing is the process of relating oneself to the external world, both the interpersonal world and the world of inanimate objects, and is predicated on the capacity to distinguish between inner and outer reality. The STIPO assesses reality testing in terms of depersonalization, perception of bodily sensations, experience of inner and outer reality, and understanding of ones' social impact on others. Marked impairment in reality testing is reflected in hallucinatory and delusional thinking, in an inordinate orientation towards magical or supernatural experience and in fixed hypochondriacal ideas that have a delusional quality.

Marked impairment in reality testing distinguishes patients with atypical psychoses from those falling into the borderline level of organization. The presence of mild or transient impairment of reality testing can be characteristic of the borderline level of organization and, when present, will distinguish the borderline from the neurotic and normal groups.

Examples for questions assessing Reality Testing are:

- *"Are there times when you have a sense you are not your usual self, or that you are so disconnected from your usual experience that you feel estranged from yourself and the surrounding world?"* (Dissociation)
- *"Have you had the experience of feeling detached from yourself, of either watching yourself from outside like you were watching a film about you doing something or perhaps having the experience of a part of your body being either not attached to you or non-existent?"* (Depersonalization)

2.1.4 *Structure and analysis of the STIPO*

After a brief introductory information about the interview (screening questions for other diagnoses, important life events like hospitalizations, break-ups etc.) the STIPO is conducted in the given order across the seven domains. The results from these seven domains form a personality profile and provide the basis for the overall structural diagnosis.

Scoring on item-level

The STIPO consists of 94 items which are scored by the interviewer while it is administered. Each item is rated on a 0-2 scale, with "0" reflecting the absence of pathology in the characteristic being assessed by a given question, "2" reflecting the clear presence of pathology in the characteristic being assessed, and a score of "1" representing an intermediate status in which some pathology in the characteristic being assessed is reflected in the response.

Domain scores calculated by mean-of-items

Scores for each STIPO domain and subscale are calculated by averaging the 0-2 scores for the items in that particular domain or subscale. The psychometric qualities of the scores on item-level have been examined by Stern and colleagues (2007).

Domain scores through 5-point rating scales

In addition to the calculation of item-based domain and subscale scores by taking the mean of items in that domain or subscale, the interviewer also completes a 5-point clinical rating for each domain, and several additional subscales of the interview. The 5-point scales define the range of health and pathology for each section being rated (1 indicating absence of pathology, 5 indicating severe pathology in the specific domain). For example, an examinee with a score of 1 on the Quality of Object Relations Scale would have described, across the various questions in the Object Relations section of the interview, strong, enduring and satisfying object relations, not viewed in terms of need fulfillment, and would demonstrate the ability to combine sexuality and intimacy. In contrast, an examinee with a score of 5 on the same scale would have described a severe paucity of attachments, a view of relationships based strictly on need fulfillment, little capacity for empathy, and little to no capacity to sustain interest or commitment to others across time.

The 5-point scales are rated by the interviewer after the last question in a given section has been administered. The interviewer is instructed to use his or her clinical impression of the examinee, based on responses to STIPO questions, the examinee's non-verbal behavior during the interview, and the interviewer's clinical sense of the examinee, bearing in mind factors that appear evident during the interview but that might not be manifest in the examinee's verbal responses. Also, in contrast to the mean-of-items scoring method, in which each STIPO item is given equal weight in the mean score, the 5-point clinical ratings allow the interviewer, based on his or her clinical judgment, to differentially weight items within a given domain when assigning the 5-point rating.

As the item-based scoring system has been investigated elsewhere (Stern et al., 2007), the focus of this study is to examine the validity of the clinical 5-point ratings by investigating the usefulness of a prototype of BPO based on these 5-point ratings.

Profiling personality organization

Using these clinical 5-point ratings, the interviewer can construct a profile of personality organization of the subject, based on the seven domains. The three primary domains of Identity, Primitive Defenses and Reality Testing are used to make a structural diagnosis as described by Kernberg (1984). Patients can be classified as falling into normal, neurotic or borderline range of organization. Based on the STIPO dimensional ratings, this categorization can be made, differentiating normal, neurotic and borderline personality organization. The detailed descriptions of the profiles are described in the STIPO manual (Clarkin et al., 2004) and are summarized in table 3.

Table 3. STIPO dimensional clinical ratings across the different levels of personality structure

STIPO Domain	Normal	Neurotic 1	Neurotic 2	Borderline 1	Borderline 2	Borderline 3
Identity	1	1	2	3	4	5
Object Relations	1	2	2, 3	3	4	5
Primitive Defenses	1	1	2	3	4	5
Coping/Rig.	1	2	3	3, 4	4, 5	4, 5
Aggression	1	2	2	3	3, 4	5
Moral values	1	2	2, 3	2, 3	2, 3	5
Reality Testing	1	1, 2	1, 2, 3	2, 3	2, 3, 4	3, 4

Note: 1 = absence of pathology, 5= very severe pathology

Subjects falling into normal and neurotic 1 group have consolidated identity, show no use of primitive defenses or disturbance in reality testing. Patients falling into Neurotic 2 group have some degree of superficiality in sense of self and/or others and might show some use primitive defenses. Patients located at borderline level of personality organization are divided according to severity of pathology into BP1, BP2, BP3. Ranging from BP1 to BP3, levels of identity diffusion, use of primitive defense mechanisms and aggression and disturbance of object relations and of morality increase. Essentially, lower scores indicate lower pathology and higher scores indicate higher pathology.

In figure 2, a STIPO personality profile shows the seven domains and subdomains on the horizontal axis, while the vertical axis indicates the dimensional rating of severity. Both scoring systems are reflected in the profile, the solid line presenting the clinical 5-point ratings and the dotted line the mean-of-items. The latter was transformed from the 3-point scale (0,1,2) to a 5-point scale (1-5) to enable comparability in the graphic illustration. This patient is located at the level of BP2, as most of the scores were rated with a score of 4 (especially Identity, Object Relations and Primitive Defenses).

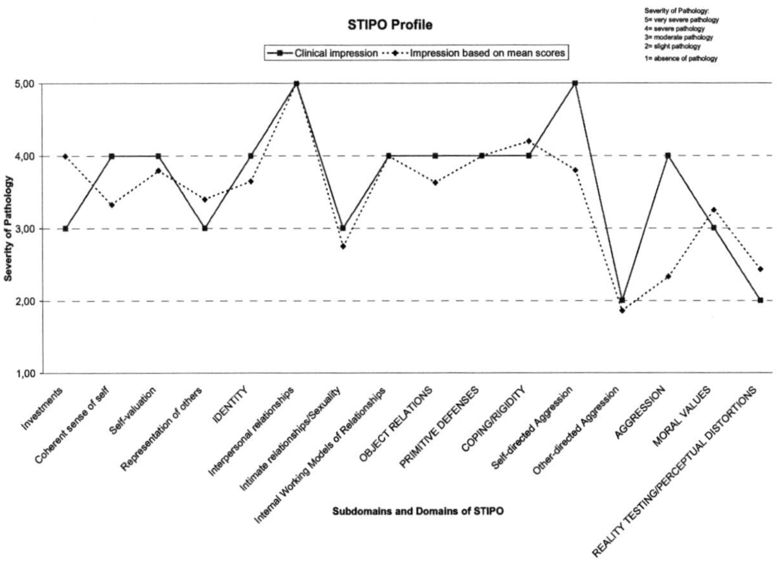

Figure 2. *STIPO profile of Personality Organization*

2.2. <u>Inventory of Personality Organization</u>

The *Inventory of Personality Organization* (IPO; Clarkin, Foelsch, & Kernberg, 2001; Foelsch et al., 2000) is an 83-item self-report instrument that assesses the three major dimensions relevant to Kernberg's model of personality organization as well as two other supplementary scales (i.e., moral values, aggression). The IPO is intended to aid in the assessment of the behaviors and psychological features reflective of identity diffusion, primitive psychological defenses and reality testing in both clinical and nonclinical populations.

Prior research (Lenzenweger et al., 2001) has demonstrated that each of the three primary scales Reality Testing, Primitive Defenses and Identity Diffusion displayed acceptable internal consistency (α in a range from .79 to .88) and good test-retest reliability (Identity diffusion: r=.78; Primitive defenses: r=.72; Reality Testing: r= .73) in a non-clinical sample. Also, item-level confirmatory factor analysis supported a two-factor latent structure as well as a three-factor latent structure of the IPO, both consistent with Kernberg's model of Borderline Personality Organization (1984; 1996), that is Reality Testing vs. Primitive Defenses- Identity Diffusion. The two-factor model is seen as representing the latent structure of the IPO most efficiently, consistent with Kernberg's model which emphasizes the close link between primitive defenses and identity diffusion in severe personality pathology and a well-demarcated reality testing process, separate from the identity diffusion and primitive defense processes. Lenzenweger and colleagues (2001) also examined the basic criterion validity of the IPO by observing the IPO in relation to positive affect, negative affect and aggressive dyscontrol. The three primary scales of the IPO were associated with higher levels of negative affect, irritability, dysphoria as well as lower levels of positive affect. Also, the IPO Reality Testing scale was closely related to various measures of psychotic-like phenomena.

Sum scores and mean scores for each of the five scales of the IPO are based on 83 items, each on a scale ranging from "(1) Never True" to "(5) Always True". Higher scores indicate more pathology in the respective domain. The IPO was included in this study primarily to investigate the incremental validity of the STIPO over this self-report precursor. A high overlap between the self-report and the interview measure is expected, for example in the scales Identity diffusion or Primitive Defenses. The results from the five IPO domains can be compared to the results from the corresponding STIPO domains.

2.3. Schedule for Nonadaptive and Adaptive Personality

The *Schedule for Nonadaptive and Adaptive Personality* (SNAP; Clark, 1993; Clark et al., 2005) is a factor analytically derived self-report questionnaire designed to assess trait dimensions important in the domain of personality disorders. Based on a dimensional model of personality, it attempts to identify those traits that are pertinent to both the normal range and the pathological range of personality. It was developed by having clinicians sort personality-relevant symptoms into synonym categories, then reducing these categories further by combining symptom clusters that were highly correlated with one another. The final instrument consists of 375 true/false items and is composed of 15 scales: 12 trait scales assess specific or primary traits and 3 temperament scales measure more general affective traits. It also provides 5 validity scales and an overall validity index to identify profiles that may be invalid owing to carelessness, defensiveness, answer patterns due to social desirability, acquiescence or deviance. In SNAP, 13 diagnostic scales assessing the personality disorder criteria according to the DSM-III-R (American Psychiatric

Association, 1987) are included, SNAP-2 (Clark et al., 2005) includes diagnostic scales according to the DSM-IV (American Psychiatric Association, 1994). Table 4 shows the SNAP scales, the Trait and Temperament scales in the first column, validity scales in the second and diagnostic scales in the third.

Table 4. SNAP Scales

Trait and Temperament Scales	**Validity Scales**	**Diagnostic Scales**
Negative Temperament	Variable Response Inconsistency	Paranoid
Mistrust	Deviance	Schizoid
Manipulativeness	True Response Inconsistency	Schizotypal
Aggression	Rare Virtues	Antisocial
Self-harm	Desirable Response Inconsistency	Borderline
Eccentric Perceptions	Invalidity Index	Histrionic
Dependency		Narcissistic
Positive Temperament		Avoidant
Exhibitionism		Dependent
Entitlement		Obsessive-Compulsive
Detachment		Passive-Aggressive
Disinhibition		Sadistic
Impulsivity		Self-Defeating
Propriety		
Workaholism		

The SNAP Trait Temperament Scales showed very good convergent validity in comparison to other questionnaires aimed at traits associated with personality disorders (Clark et al., 1993; 1996; Reynolds & Clark, 2001). The SNAP Validity Scales also proved good convergent and discriminant validity, especially for the Rare Virtues and Deviance scales (Simms & Clark, 2001). The SNAP Diagnostic Scales demonstrated strong convergent validity with interview measures, in particular with the SIDP-R (Pfohl et al., 1989), showing a median convergent validity coefficient of .54, which is considerably higher than that found in previous studies using other self-report instruments and/or interviews. Discriminant correlations were also good but lower than the convergent correlations, probably reflecting the problem of comorbidity in personality disorder diagnoses (Clark, 1993). Also, very good 9-month test-retest reliability for the Diagnostic Scales could be demonstrated, ranging from .58 to .81, and good results for the predictive validity were found (Melley, Oltmanns & Turkheimer, 2002). Further research has shown that the SNAP scales distinguish patients with personality disorders from a variety of comparison groups, including normal individuals and other clinical samples. An association between core temperament scales with specific personality disorders was seen, for example the subscales "Self-Harm" and "Aggression" were related to BPD, whereas other Temperament scales (e.g. "Negative Affect", "Detachment") seemed to be associated to the presence of personality pathology in general (Morey et al., 2003).

Respondents fill out the 375 items, replying "yes" or "no" to each item. The number of items endorsed for each scale is counted, yielding the raw score. Both raw scores and T-scores are available for all scales (validity, trait and temperament, diagnostic). The diagnostic scales consist of items which are similar to the DSM- criteria and a certain number of criteria is needed to assign a personality disorder diagnosis. Each personality disorder criterion is represented by at least two items. The number of items needed to meet each specific criterion varies. Clark (1993) provided two scoring methods for these scales. A criterion-based method can be used to assign dichotomous diagnoses. Using this method, it is necessary to determine whether the person endorsed the required number of SNAP items for each personality disorder criterion, and then to compute the number of criteria that are met for each personality disorder diagnosis. A dimensional score can also be obtained by counting the total number of items that are endorsed for each personality disorder scale (regardless of which criteria the items represent). Clark recommends the latter approach because dimensional scores are more reliable and also correlated more strongly and systematically with interview based diagnostic ratings. In this study, the criterion-based method was chosen only for the computation of the personality disorder frequencies in the sample. For the remaining quantitative analysis and single case studies, the dimensional method was used to evaluate the level of SNAP personality pathology in relation to pathology assessed by the STIPO or the other self-report measures.

2.4. Inventory of Interpersonal Problems – Personality Disorders Scales

The *Inventory of Interpersonal Problems – Personality Disorders Scales* (IIP-PD; Pilkonis et al., 1996) was developed based on the items of the *Inventory of Interpersonal Problems* (Horowitz et al., 1988) in an effort to find a brief self-report screening tool to identify individuals with personality disorder diagnoses. It is a 28-item screening index for the presence or absence of a personality disorder, which has proven effective both in clinical and in nonclinical populations (Pilkonis et al., 1996; Scarpa et al., 1999; Stern et al., 2000). Factor analyses have shown a three-factor solution fitting the data best. The first factor contained 11 items and was named "interpersonal sensitivity" because of the strong affectivity and reactivity that the items suggested, for example "I am too sensitive to rejection", " It is hard for me to ignore criticism from other people". The second factor, named "Interpersonal ambivalence" contained 10 items and included statements suggesting a struggle against others and an inability to join collaboratively in either work or love. Examples are " It is hard to accept another person's authority over me", "It is hard to be supportive of another person's goals in life". The third factor, consisting of seven items, was labelled "aggression" because of the active, hostile content of the items like "I argue with other people too much" or " I am too aggressive toward other people". Two additional scales consisting of nineteen items were also identified as being useful in discriminating between individuals who met criteria for a Cluster C diagnosis and those who did not.

The initial validation study (Pilkonis et al., 1996) conducted with a psychiatric patient sample showed that the 28 item IIP Scale has good operating characteristics, in particular good positive predictive power (PPP; >.85) and high sensitivity in distinguishing individuals with or without a personality disorder diagnosis. The ability to discriminate between cluster B and C disorders was more limited, due to Cluster B patients also endorsing items associated with Cluster C disorders. Further analysis of the 47 personality disorder scale items conducting a confirmatory factor analysis (CFA) found that a hierarchical model showed the best fit, with one second-order factor and five first-order factors, supporting the hypothesis of a single latent construct reflecting general personality dysfunction (Kim, Pilkonis & Barkham, 1997; Stern et al., 2000).

The utility of the IIP-PD in screening for the presence or absence of a personality disorder was shown in nonclinical samples, confirming that individuals who exceeded the DSM symptom threshold for at least one personality disorder rarely scored above the IIP-PD cutoff. The cutoff score is computed as the mean score of all 28 items, each rated on a 0 ("not at all") to 4 ("extremely") scale. A cutoff of 1.1 was considered to provide the greatest diagnostic and clinical utility (Stern et al., 2000). In this study, this instrument was included as an important indicator of personality pathology and the cutoff at 1.1 was chosen, aiming at high specificity when identifying any versus no personality disorder in the sample.

2.5. Big Five Inventory

The *Big Five Inventory* (BFI-44) by John, Donahue & Kentle (1991) is a 44-item self-report instrument assessing the "Big Five" personality dimensions. The Five-Factor-Model (FFM) is a lexically derived dimensional model of personality and includes the domains of "Neuroticism" (negative affectivity), "Extraversion" (positive affectivity), "Conscientiousness" (constraint), "Openness" (unconventionality) and "Agreeableness" versus "Antagonism" (Costa & McCrae, 1992a; Costa & McCrae, 1990; Widiger & Costa, Jr., 1994). These five domains can each further be differentiated into six underlying facets within each domain. For example, Costa and McCrae (1995) suggested that the domain of "Agreeableness" could be usefully differentiated into more specific facets of trust, straightforwardness, altruism, compliance, modesty and tendermindedness. The FFM has proven important in assessing personality traits both in normal as well as clinical samples and has been examined in its utility to describe personality disorders. For example, Widiger and colleagues (Widiger et al., 1994) suggested how each of the 10 DSM-IV personality disorders might be described in terms of the domains and facets of the FFM, as conceptualized by Costa and McCrae (1995). Trull and colleagues (2003) examined the relationship of BPD to the FFM by developing a prototype of BPD and examining its association with measures of BPD. They concluded that BPD can be considered a maladaptive variant of FFM personality traits. The BFI-44 was included in this study in order to examine the incremental validity of the theory-based BPO prototype over the lexically derived FFM and also to inspect in the single case section how the results of this FFM measure relate to the other instruments.

The BFI-44 was constructed to allow efficient and flexible assessment of the five dimensions of the FFM when there is no need for more differentiated measurement of the facets (which are the subordinate dimensions of each of the five factors). The items were selected from Big Five prototype definitions that had been developed through expert ratings and subsequent factor analytic verification in observer personality ratings. The 44 items are brief descriptions of traits, for example when assessing the item "original" from the domain openness, the respondent is asked to choose how much he agrees to the item "is original, comes up with new ideas". John, Donahue and Kentle (1991) report that the reliabilities of the BFI-44 compare to the longer version NEO-FFI (Costa & McCrae, 1992b) and that convergence correlations for the scales from these two instruments are substantial.

2.6. Positive and Negative Affect Schedule

The *Positive and Negative Affect Schedule –Expanded Form* (PANAS-X) by Watson, Clark and Harkness (1994) was used to examine several dimensions of positive and negative affect important in the diagnosis of patients with and without personality disorders. The PANAS-X is the expanded form of the PANAS (Watson, Clark & Tellegen, 1988), a 20-item measure assessing the two major dimensions of normative emotion, namely positive affect (enthusiasm, activeness, alertness) and negative affect (aversive mood states, including anger, guilt, fear, nervousness, contempt). The primary concern during the development of the scale was to select descriptors that were relatively pure markers of either Negative Affect or Positive Affect; that is, terms that had a substantial loading on one factor but a near-zero loading on the other (Watson, Clark & Harkness, 1994). The 60-item PANAS-X consists of two general dimension scales (i.e. positive affect, negative affect), four basic negative emotion scales (fear, hostility, guilt, sadness), three basic positive emotion scales (joviality, self-assurance, attentiveness) and four scales assessing other affective states (shyness, fatigue, serenity, surprise). The PANAS-X yields dimensional scores for the higher order (i.e. positive affect, negative affect) and lower order scales and can be used for assessment of short-term, state affect as well as for measuring long-term individual differences in affect.

Watson, Clark and Harkness (1994) report that internal consistencies range from .36 to .90 for positive affect and from .79 to .93 for negative affect, depending

on temporal instructions. Different temporal instructions are offered in order to assess state or trait positive and negative affectivity (i.e. instructions can refer either to "at the moment", "today", "past week days", "weeks" or "generally"). In this study, patients were asked to rate themselves on the items on the basis how they felt in the past few weeks, utilizing the instrument as a state measure. The 2-month test-retest stability of the PANAS for the "past-few-weeks" assessment of positive affect is .43, for negative affect .41 and for the lower order scales ranges from .23 (Surprise) to. 49 (Shyness).
The PANAS-X was employed to investigate the levels of positive and negative affect in relation to personality pathology, and also to illustrate the different facets of positive and negative affect when examining the single cases.

2.7. Buss-Durkee-Inventory

The well-known *Buss-Durkee-Inventory* (Buss & Durkee, 1957) was used to assess different kinds of hostility. The inventory consists of eight subscales: "Assault", "Indirect Hostility", "Irritability" and "Verbal Hostility" defining Buss and Durkee's second or "behavioral" factor, whereas the subscales "Negativism", "Resentment", "Suspicion" and "Guilt" are regarded as "attitudinal" subscales. 75 items are given in the true-false format and yield sum scores for each scale. The hostility items were scaled for social desirability , and social desirability was correlated with probability of endorsement, resulting in rather low r's of .27 and .30 for college men and women, seeming to reflect the item construction techniques in the present study (Buss & Durkee, 1957).
This scale was included to examine different aspects of hostility and negative attitude, expecting these to be important in diagnosing and differentiating patients with personality disorders, in particular BPO patients, from other patient groups. Also, the association of these hostility scales to negative affect is of interest, following Lenzenweger and colleagues' results (2001), who found BPO-typical scales of the IPO associated both with negative affect and with aggressive dyscontrol (operationalized as the Buss Durkee subscale "Irritability").

2.8. Brief Symptom Inventory

The BSI (Derogatis, 1993) is a self-report measure which consists of 53 items and yields one global score of distress, the global severity index. The BSI also provides scaled scores on nine symptom patterns: anxiety, somatization, obsessive-compulsive, interpersonal sensitivity, depression, hostility, phobic anxiety, paranoid ideation, and psychoticism. Individuals respond to the items using a five-point scale that has anchors at "not at all" (1) to "extremely" (5). According to Derogatis (1993), internal consistency (coefficient alpha) for the nine symptom patterns ranges from .71 (psychoticism) to .85 (depression). The test-retest reliability for the nine scales range from .68 (somatization) to .91 (phobic anxiety) with a mean of .82 (Derogatis, 1993).

The BSI contains the following nine primary symptom sub-scales. The scale "Somatisation" reflects distress arising from perceptions of bodily dysfunction. The dimension "Obsessive compulsive" focuses on thoughts, impulses and actions that are experienced as unremitting and irresistible by the individual, but are of an unwanted nature. "Interpersonal sensitivity" centers on feeling of personal inadequacy, inferiority and self-doubt. The symptoms of the "depression" dimension reflect a representative range of the indicators of clinical depression . General signs such as nervousness and tension are included in the dimension "Anxiety", for example feelings of apprehension, panic attacks and feelings of terror. The dimension "Hostility" includes thoughts, feelings, or actions that are characteristic of the negative affect state of anger. "Phobic anxiety" is defined as a persistent fear response to a specific person, place, object or situation that is irrational disproportionate to the stimulus and leads to avoidance or escape behavior. The dimension "paranoid ideation" represents paranoid behavior fundamentally as a disordered mode of thinking. The cardinal characteristics of projective thought, hostility, suspiciousness, grandiosity, centrality fear of loss of autonomy and delusions are viewed as primarily aspects of this disorder. Finally, the scale "Psychoticism" was developed to represent the construct of psychoticism as a continuous dimension of human experience. Items indicative of a withdrawn, isolated schizoid lifestyle were included, as were first-rank symptoms of schizophrenia, such as thought control. This scale provided for a graduated continuum from mild interpersonal alienation to dramatic psychosis.

The BSI scales were included to assess axis-I symptoms and to inspect the relation of axis I pathology to personality pathology in the total sample and in the single cases.

3 Data Analysis

The statistical analysis was done with SPSS for Windows (Version 12.0). The data was analyzed to describe demographics, range and statistics of STIPO domain scores, SNAP diagnoses, BSI and GAF scores.

All variables used to examine hypotheses 1 through 5 were on interval scale level.

In a first step, a BPO similarity index was computed. For this purpose, the STIPO domain scores of the prototypical profile were compared to each patient's actual STIPO scores on the same variables to obtain a BPO similarity index, reflecting the similarity between the expert prototypical profile and the individual STIPO scores. The squared Euclidian distance served as a BPO similarity index[1] for each patient, which was a new dimensional variable used for the computations of hypotheses 3 through 5.

The BPO prototype's ability to discriminate between groups was examined by means of a hierarchical cluster analysis. The cluster solution produced from the hierarchical cluster analysis was tested by also conducting a nonhierarchical k-means cluster analysis. The resulting clusters, following hypothesis 1, were evaluated with regard to group differences in general functioning, axis I pathology and axis II pathology by one-way analyses of variance. To account for different sample sizes, levene tests on homogeneity of variances were conducted. In the case of heterogenic variances ($p < .05$), the Welch Statistic with subsequent Games-Howell post-hoc tests was chosen. If variances were homogeneous, ANOVA F-tests and Tukey post-hoc tests were conducted. Both post-hoc tests took into account the cumulated alpha error. All variables were tested with regard to normal distribution (Kolmogorov-Smirnov-Test; $p <.05$). For non-normally distributed variables, the results were confirmed with Kruskal-Wallis-H-Tests.

---

[1] As the Euclidian distance is conceptualized as a "dissimilarity measure", the squared Euclidian distance was multiplied with (-1) to yield a "similarity index". Computations based on this "similarity index" will be presented for ease of reading.

The second hypothesis, examining the interrater reliability of the 5-point ratings of the four prototypical domains, was computed by examining the intraclass correlation coefficients (ICCs; Shrout & Fleiss, 1979).

Following hypothesis 3, the convergent validity of the BPO similarity index was tested by computing bivariate correlations between the BPO similarity index and measures of axis II pathology. As not all variables were normally distributed (tested with Kolmogorov-Smirnov-Test; $p < .05$), Spearman correlations were computed between the BPO similarity index and these variables from the self-report instruments.

Finally, in hypotheses 4 and 5, the incremental validity of the BPO similarity index was tested by computing hierarchical regression analyses. In testing the incremental validity of the BPO index over the Five Factor Model of personality, hierarchical regression analyses were computed with the BFI-44 as first factor and the BPO similarity index as second factor and various axis II symptoms and correlates as dependent variables. Similarly, in hypothesis 5; the incremental validity of the BPO similarity index over the IPO was examined by computing hierarchical regression analyses with the IPO as first factor and the BPO index as second factor as well as the various axis II symptoms and correlates as dependent variables. An alpha level of .05 was used for all statistical tests.

V RESULTS

1 Quantitative Analysis : Examination of the total sample

1.1. Sample description

1.1.1 Demographic data

The number of participating subjects was N=60. This was the remaining group of patients who agreed to participate and who also completed both parts of the assessment, the interview and the self-report measures. In total, 86 subjects had been asked to participate: 20 of these were not interested in the study, four patients refused to be videotaped, one dropped out after the interview and did not fill out the questionnaires and one patient dropped out during the interview because of difficulties in understanding the questions.

Of the 60 patients, 41 (68%) were female, 19 (32%) were male and the age ranged from 18 to 55 years, with a mean age of 31 years. As table 5 shows, 15 (25%) of these patients were recruited from private practice, seven (11,7%) from the outpatient department of NYPH, two (3,3%) from the day program and the majority of 36 patients (60%) came from the inpatient unit.

Table 5. Treatment modality

	N	Percent
private practice	15	25.0
outpatient department	7	11.7
day program	2	3.3
inpatient unit	36	60.0
Total	60	100.0

As for the patients' relationship status, 52 (86,7 %) were single and eight patients (13,3 %) were married. In the past year, 23 of the patients (38,3%) were in no relationship, 18 (30%) patients spent between one and ten months in a romantic relationship, and 19 patients (31,7%) spent the complete last year in a relationship. Being in a relationship included the option "being married".

The level of education is shown in table 6. Seven (11,7%) had less than high school education, 24 patients (40%) had a high school diploma, and 23 patients (38,3 %) had a college degree.

Table 6. *Education*

	N	Percent
less than high school	7	11.7
high school or GED	24	40.0
associates / some college	3	5.0
Bachelors	15	25.0
Masters	8	13.3
Missing	3	5.0
Total	60	100.0

As for the employment situation, the vast majority of 40 (67%) patients did not work at the time of the assessment. Eleven (18%) subjects worked part-time and nine (15%) worked full-time. Considering that many of the patients were long-term inpatients, the information about the situation regarding work and education in the past five year was considered as well. Regarding the primary role in the past five years, 17 (28,3 %) of the 60 patients worked primarily, six (10,0 %) were primarily students, 35 (58,3 %) were involved in both, and two (3,3 %) in neither. Of course, this information does not take into account how much of this time the subjects were actually working or studying, but does provide an overview of the primary area in which the patients were involved.

1.1.2 STIPO domains

The results from the STIPO can best be shown in a patient profile as in figure 2. As one of the main objectives of this study is to discriminate between different patient groups through a STIPO-based prototype and as separate patient groups and their STIPO results will be examined more detail later, for now the descriptive results of the total sample in the seven STIPO domains will be presented.

As illustrated when introducing the structure of the STIPO (section IV. 2.1.4.), two different scores can be obtained per STIPO domain. The first is the item-based score which is the mean of the 0, 1, 2 scores for each of the items per domain. For example, in the domain "Primitive Defenses" the mean consists of the scores of the nine items "Paranoia", "Erratic behavior", "Idealization / devaluation" etc. In these mean scores, each item is weighted equally. In contrast to this, in the second scoring system, a clinical rating is given for the overall domain, in this case "Primitive Defenses", on a scale from 1 to 5. This

score, ranging from (1) "absence of pathology" to (5) "very severe pathology", additionally takes into account the interviewer's clinical impression.
The two scoring systems complement each other, and the descriptive data per domain is presented for both systems. The following tables show the mean scores of the sample in the seven STIPO domains, first the item-based results and then the overall clinical results. In table 7, scores of 0 indicate absence of pathology, scores of 2 indicate pathology. In table 8 the scores range from 1 (absence of pathology) to 5 (very severe pathology).

Table 7. Descriptives of the STIPO domains (mean scores of item-based ratings, 0-2 point ratings) (N= 60)

	M	SD	Min	Max
Identity	1.09	0.59	0.09	1.86
Object Relations	0.74	0.53	0.00	1.74
Primitive Defenses	0.87	0.54	0.00	1.80
Coping / Rigidity	1.21	0.49	0.00	2.00
Aggression	0.59	0.44	0.00	1.75
Moral Values	0.61	0.56	0.00	1.88
Reality Testing	0.48	0.35	0.00	1.57

M = mean, *SD* = standard deviation, *Min* = Minimum, *Max* = Maximum

Table 8. Descriptives of the STIPO domains (1-5 point overall clinical ratings) (N= 60)

	M	SD	Min	Max
Identity	3.58	1.18	1.00	5.00
Object Relations	3.18	1.07	1.00	5.00
Primitive Defenses	3.25	1.34	1.00	5.00
Coping / Rigidity	3.77	1.14	1.00	5.00
Aggression	3.05	1.29	1.00	5.00
Moral Values	2.31	1.12	1.00	5.00
Reality Testing	2.05	0.83	1.00	5.00

M = mean, *SD* = standard deviation, *Min* = Minimum, *Max* = Maximum

On an average, in both scoring procedures, the sample shows the highest pathology in "Coping and Rigidity" and the least in "Reality Testing". These overall ratings across the whole sample, of course, do not discriminate between patient groups with different levels of pathology. The differentiation between patient clusters with high and low pathology in the STIPO will be examined in context of the first hypothesis.

Of the two scoring systems, this study focuses on the clinical ratings, the 1-5 ratings. This was done in order to examine the validity of a more clinically-oriented assessment of a prototype of BPO. The computations of the BPO prototype and the following validity computations were based on the 1-5 ratings. The decision to use these ratings and not the scale mean scores (based on the 0-2 ratings) for the computations was made because the 5-point ratings were designed to identify the range of pathology in each domain on a broader scale and because the expert consensus was founded on these 5-point ratings (more details regarding the expert consensus will follow in section 1.2). To secure this decision, the correlations between the two different rating systems in each of the four prototypical domains were computed. Table 9 shows that they are reasonably high, ranging from .74 to .92 ($p < .001$).

Table 9. Correlations of the prototypical domains, assessed with the two different rating systems (item-based mean scores vs.5-point ratings) (N=60)

	1.Identity - coherence and continuity (mean of items, 0-2 pt rating)	2. Identity - Representation of others (mean of items, 0-2 pt rating)	3. Object relations (mean of items, 0-2 pt rating)	4. Object relations (mean of items, 0-2 pt rating)
1. Identity - coherence and continuity (5-point rating)	**.92 *****			
2. Identity - Representation of others (5-point rating)		**.80*****		
3. Object relations (5-point rating)			**.74*****	
4. Primitive Defenses (5-point rating)				**.86*****

* $p < .05$; ** $p < .01$; *** $p < .001$

A similarity index was computed to yield the BPO prototype, details of the method will be presented in section 1.3. This similarity index was computed both based on the 0-2 ratings as well as on the 1-5 ratings (squared Euclidian distance). The two similarity indices based on both of the scoring systems were correlated with each other, demonstrating a high correlation at .92 ($p < .001$). Thus, due to these high inter-correlations, in the quantitative analysis only the similarity index based on the 5-point ratings will be examined.

1.1.3 ***Measures of axis II pathology, GAF and BSI***

Of the seven self-report instruments that were used in the study, for now only the results of the sample as a whole in the SNAP personality disorder scales and in the IIP-PD will be shown as they are most important for establishing the validity of the STIPO scales. The instruments assessing temperamental and affective aspects (SNAP Temperament scales, BFI-44, PANAS, Buss-Durkee Scale) will not be presented descriptively, as they will be shown exemplarily in the section describing single cases (V.2.) and as they are not the focus of this study.

When scoring the SNAP personality disorders scales, a criterion-based categorical assessment as well as a dimensional scoring method can be chosen (Clark, 1993). The criterion-based score is analogous to the DSM criterion process, that is a sufficient amount of criteria is needed to meet a diagnosis. For example, to meet the diagnosis borderline personality disorder assessed with the SNAP, subjects have to fulfill five out of eight criteria (SNAP is based on DSM-III), which are assessed through several items throughout the SNAP questionnaire. The dimensional scoring method involves counting the total number of items fulfilled for each scale, regardless of which criteria the items represent, to a sum score and transforming this into (sex-specific) T-Scores in order to decide about whether the diagnosis is met. The dimensional scoring method was used in the single case section (V.2) further on. For descriptive purposes and taking into account the need for clear cut-offs when looking at a large unisex sample, the criterion-based score was used to assess the frequencies of the respective personality disorders.

Table 10. Frequencies of patients meeting criteria for SNAP personality disorders (N= 60)

	N	Percent
Paranoid PD	9	15.00
Schizoid PD	4	6.70
Schizotypal PD	5	8.30
Antisocial PD	4	6.70
Borderline PD	15	25.00
Narcissistic PD	3	5.00
Histrionic PD	6	10.00
Avoidant PD	24	40.00
Dependent PD	15	25.00
Obsessive-Compulsive PD	8	13.30

Table 10 shows that the most frequent personality disorder in this sample was avoidant personality disorder (40%), followed by borderline personality disorder (25%) and dependent personality disorder (25%). There was a high comorbidity among the personality disorders. This was assessed by counting the numbers of personality disorders each patient obtained according to the SNAP. The average number of personality disorders the patients met criteria for was 1.5. From table 11 it becomes clear that two thirds of the patients fulfilled the diagnosis for a personality disorder: 31.7% met criteria for one personality disorder and 35% for two to six personality disorders, whereas 33.3 % of the patients did not fulfill criteria for any personality disorder.

Table 11. Number of SNAP personality disorders per patient (N= 60)

	N	Percent
No personality disorder	20	33.3
1 personality disorder	19	31.7
2 personality disorders	8	13.3
3 personality disorders	5	8.3
4 personality disorders	4	6.7
5 personality disorders	2	3.3
6 personality disorders	2	3.3
Total	60	100

When inspecting the most frequent personality disorders for comorbid personality disorders, it can be seen that patients who met criteria for BPD also met criteria for avoidant personality disorder in 53% of the cases, for dependent personality disorder in 53% and for paranoid personality disorder in 33%. Similarly, patients who met criteria for avoidant personality disorder also met criteria for dependent personality disorder in 42% of the cases, for BPD in 33%. Finally, patients meeting criteria for dependent personality disorder also were diagnosed with avoidant personality disorder in 67% and with BPD in 53% of the cases.

Another important screening instrument assessing the presence or absence of personality pathology is the IIP-PD. Of the 60 patients, 39 patients (65%) described a sufficient amount of personality pathology to lie above the cut-off for a personality disorder, whereas 20 patients (33.3%) fell below the cut-off for a personality disorder (one patient did not complete this questionnaire).

With regard to the general assessment of functioning scale (GAF), due to missing data, only 47 patients (78%) of the sample can be considered. The mean score lay at 51.5 (SD 19.6), with a range from 20 to 85. Another source of information about the severity of symptoms the patients reported is the "General Severity Index" (GSI) scale of the Brief Symptom Inventory (BSI). This scale provides information on how the patient generally feels with regard to several symptom clusters like somatization, obsessive-compulsiveness, depression or anxiety. The group mean for the GSI is at 1.36 (corresponding to a T-score of 80 based on a male sample, or a T-Score of 69 based on a female sample), ranging from 0 to 3.66. This broad range of scores obviously reflects the heterogeneity of the sample. The BSI results will be discussed in greater detail in the section describing single cases (V.2.).

1.2. Expert consensus on a prototype of BPO

The first step in the development and validation of a prototype of BPO was asking the experts on BPO to find a theory-based consensus on the important elements of the prototypical profile of Borderline Personality Organization. The method for developing a prototypical BPO profile was based on the model of Lynam and Widiger (2001), who used an expert consensus approach to describe the 10 DSM-IV personality disorder's on the basis of FFM Descriptions (Likert Scales). Different from the procedure of Lynam and Widiger, who included the ratings of a large group of experts in the field of personality disorders, we decided to employ only the two raters most familiar with the theoretical model being tested in this study, that is, Kernberg's theory of personality organization (Dr. O. Kernberg and Dr. E. Caligor). Whereas in the study by Lynam and Widiger, a larger number of experts were consulted in an attempt to derive consensus regarding the relation between axis II conditions and a set of variables, which were not chosen according to any specific theory, we argue that in our study a very small group of experts is sufficient and necessary, that is, only those with the highest level of knowledge regarding the specific theory being tested in the prototype. In the case of the BPO prototype, consulting experts less familiar with the theory would result in a heterogeneity that would be less useful in the development of the BPO prototype.

For the purpose of finding the expert-consensus on the BPO prototype, I met regularly with the two experts individually to discuss which STIPO domains they each regarded relevant and crucial for a prototype of BPO. Then, I integrated their opinions on which domains to include. They were instructed to select domains according to the goal of finding a STIPO derived prototypical profile of Borderline Personality Organization (BPO) which contrasted to Neurotic Personality Organization (NPO) and thus discriminated well between BPO and NPO patients. The experts were asked to choose from any of the STIPO domains, including both the overall domains, for example "Identity", "Object Relations", "Primitive Defenses", "Coping Strategies", as well as the subdomains, for example subdomains "Investments", "Sense of self" as part of the overall domain "Identity". The amount of domains to choose was not specified. They also were asked which score in the respective STIPO domains, based on the 5-point dimensional ratings, might provide a cut-off to discriminate between NPO and BPO. For example, in the domain Primitive Defenses, would a score of 3 be regarded as NPO or BPO? The decision the experts made regarding the cut-offs will be shown when describing the individual domains.

In the following, all of the STIPO domains and subdomains will be listed and the decision the two experts made regarding inclusion or exclusion will be described. They agreed upon the relevant domains for the prototype, in part using the overall domains and in part the subdomains of the seven domains that are assessed through the STIPO. The decision was made to partially choose the scores of the subdomains instead of the overall score, for example using the subdomain “Sense of self” as part of the overall domain “Identity” instead of the domain score per se for the following reasons: the particular subdomains provide a very specific, clearly defined description, in this case of identity, and provide an internal, intrapsychic focus, in contrast to behavioral aspects. Generally, the decision was made to exclude behavioral aspects, for example the investments subdomain, from the prototype, as they are expected to less reliably discriminate between the different types of personality organization, and might distort the overall score. Behavioral aspects reflect the personality structure, but intrapsychic aspects are more likely to discriminate between different levels of personality structure. For example, both neurotic and narcissistic patients might show stable commitment to work and education, which can be regarded as behavioral aspects of the identity domain, but they can diverge at the level of identity diffusion, which is one of the intrapsychic aspects of the area of identity.

Identity

Based on the theoretical assumptions, within the domain „Identity“, individuals with BPO are expected to demonstrate variable degrees of identity pathology, as opposed to a consolidated identity in individuals with NPO. Individuals with Borderline Personality Organization should show some evidence of identity diffusion, other than a small degree of superficiality in view of others or the use of narcissistic defenses often observed in neurotic patients. There is one caveat: neurotic patients with narcissistic defenses must be carefully discriminated from healthy narcissists who present no instability in the representation of self, but have a strongly superficial sense of others, also have limitations in the capacity for empathy and therefore an overall deficit in the representation of others.

The subdomain *Investments* is assumed not to discriminate between NPO and BPO, as the presence of investments will not necessarily rule out identity diffusion. Also, too much diversity is expected within the different areas of investment across the range of patients and therefore this subcategory will not be included in the prototype.

The Subdomain *Sense of self – coherence and continuity* is regarded a good marker of identity diffusion. In all patients with BPO, severe disturbance in perceiving themselves as stable and consistent across situations and time is expected. Also describing themselves fully and integrated, both with negative as well as positive aspects, is anticipated to be a source of difficulty for BPO patients. We expect different intensities in problems of self versus object descriptions. For example a narcissistic patient might be able to provide a good description of himself, but a bad description of others, whereas a schizoid patient might give a bad self description, but a detailed description of others; however, overall we expect all BPO patients to show a considerable amount of pathology in this domain. Thus, a score of 3 or higher should indicate the presence of BPO as opposed to a score of 1 or 2 indicating NPO.

The Subdomain *Self valuation* is not expected to discriminate well between BPO and NPO, for example because a person with neurotic personality organization can, similarly to a person located at borderline organization, have a high score demonstrating narcissistic defenses.

Representation of others is anticipated to discriminate well between BPO and NPO patients. Patients at the level of BPO are thought to have difficulties in reflective functioning, in seeing others as whole objects, in describing them in a full and nuanced manner, and in reflecting on the personality of others beyond immediate behavior. Also, we expect BPO patients to have considerably more difficulties in assessing others, perceiving social cues and imagining other's thoughts and opinions of the subject than NPO patients. We anticipate clear differences between NPO, indicated by scores of 1 or 2, and BPO, scoring 3 or higher.

Object Relations

In general, object relations are compromised in patients with BPO, meaning that there should be some conflicts in interpersonal relationships, in particular in intimate relationships. Regarding the subdomains of object relations, in the subdomain *Interpersonal Relationships* we expect to find a degree of variance, ranging from clinging-dependent behavior of the obsessive-compulsive personality disorder patient to the withdrawal of the schizoid personality disorder patient. Some patients with personality disorders might experience their relations with friends and coworkers as more unsatisfactory than others, and the severity of the personality disorder might influence the severity of the impairment of this subdomain. Hence, due to the expected variability we do not expect this subdomain alone to discriminate between NPO and BPO.

The subdomain *Intimate Relationships and Sexuality* usually is particularly compromised in BPO patients, although it might vary. For example, patient with histrionic personality disorder might be very promiscuous, others might show complete inhibition, and some BPO patients also have good sexual relationships. Also because some patients located at the level of NPO might present quite some inhibition in some contexts, we do expect too many patterns for this subdomain to be able to discriminate between BPO and NPO.

Also, the subdomain *Internal Working Model of Relationships,* assessing aspects like difficulties with empathy, capacity to care about the needs of others independent of needs of the self and a sense of entitlement, is expected to be very variable across the range of borderline and neurotic personality pathology, and should, therefore, in itself not clearly differentiate between NPO and BPO.

In total, we anticipate a fair amount of variability in the quality of object relations, internal and external, across patients located at different levels of personality organization, most likely resulting in quite variable scores within the subdomains of object relations. Thus, the experts found the consensus to use the overall score of this domain, including difficulties in all areas of object relations, as well in friendships as in intimate relationships. Aiming at high specificity, a high, that is pathological score was chosen as the hypothesized cut-off between NPO and BPO. Ratings of 4 or 5 are expected to reflect BPO, whereas a score between 1 and 3 is anticipated to describe neurotic patients.

Primitive Defenses

The domain assessing the predominant style of defense mechanisms is one of the core domains expected to discriminate between levels of personality organization. Borderline Personality Organization is characterized by the predominance of primitive defensive operations centering on splitting, whereas Neurotic Personality Organization presents higher level defenses, mostly relying on repression. Thus, the domain "Primitive Defenses" is anticipated to discriminate between the different levels of personality organization; scores of 1 to 3 reflecting NPO, and 4 or 5 indicating BPO.

Coping/ Rigidity

The use of adaptive coping strategies is expected to be quite variable amongst neurotic, narcissistic patients with pervasively rigid coping strategies and borderline patients with frequently chaotic ways in dealing with stressful events and experiences. This domain will therefore not be part of the prototype. Originally, the domain Coping and Rigidity was included in the interview for discrimination between normal and pathological personality organization, which is not the focus of this study.

Aggression

The domain of aggression will not be included in the prototype as the behavioral aspect of aggression is difficult to assess. In theory primitive aggression is central to the experience of BPO, meaning that it is the behavioral manifestation of the hypothesized structural drive or impulse, but clinically it proves to be more complicated (e.g. passive-aggressive behavior). This is the reason why the domain of aggression had also not been included in the original Structural Interview.

Moral Values

The domain of Moral Values will not be included in the prototype for two reasons: It is not expected to discriminate between NPO and BPO, but only between different levels of Borderline Personality Organization which is not the focus of this study.

Reality Testing and Perceptual Distortions

Kernberg's theory suggests that the dimension Reality Testing and Perceptual Distortions should be variable across the range of borderline and neurotic personality pathology, and should, therefore, not influence the prototype. By this is meant that in both patient groups of NPO and BPO, reality testing in general is maintained, but there might be a slight degree of perceptual distortions or impairment of reality testing. As this domain is intended to discriminate between non- psychotic patients and patients located at Psychotic Personality Organization, it will not be included in the prototype.

In sum, based on the 5-point dimensional ratings of the STIPO domains and subdomains, a patient located at BPO is expected to obtain scores of :
(1) Three or greater in the Identity-subdomain "Coherent sense of self",
(2) Three or greater in the Identity-subdomain "Representation of others",
(3) Four or greater in the domain "Object Relations"; and
(4) Four or greater in the domain "Primitive Defenses".

This study aims at discrimination between NPO and BPO through a *prototype* with a high specificity and low sensitivity, that is, the patients with BPO that are captured by the prototype should be clearly low level BPO (severely disturbed), whereas the high level BPO patients might fall into the NPO cluster (risk of false negative). Commensurate with the goal of reducing false positives (high specificity), rather high scores were chosen as cut-offs in the four prototype domains. For example, a patient located at higher BPO might receive a score of 3 in Object Relations and thus be categorized as "non-prototypical", although falling into the higher level of BPO range. These theory-based cut-offs should be scrutinized in this study.

The hypothesized profile of a BPO prototype is shown in the following figure 3. The figure includes a patient's STIPO profile with the scores based on the 1-5 ratings. The four prototypical domains are marked with vertical arrows, showing the range of prototypicality in each domain. The other domains and subdomains are omitted when examining how many prototype criteria a patient meets and when assessing the patient's level of personality organization based on the prototype.

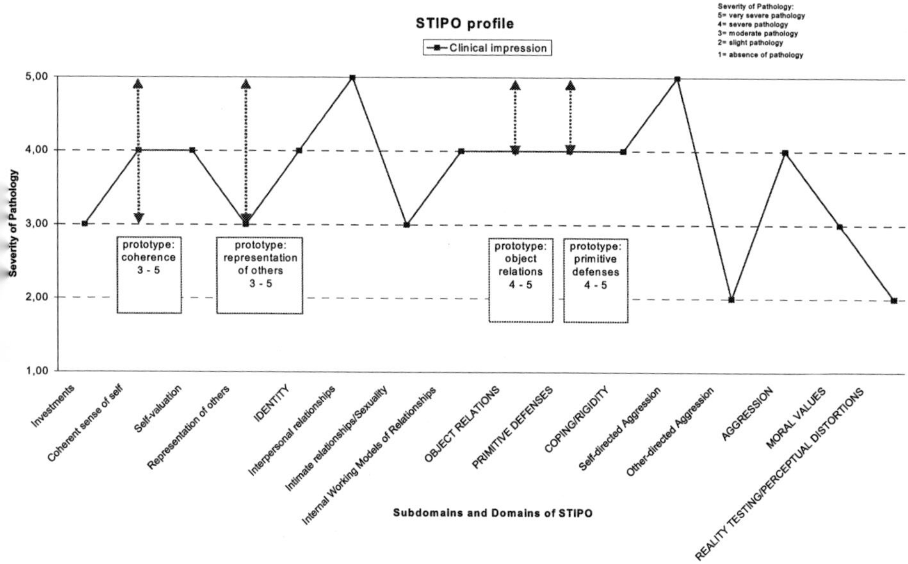

Figure 3. *STIPO profile with prototypical domains*

1.3. BPO Similarity Index

After the hypothesized prototypical profile of BPO was created, the next step was to construct a BPO similarity index. For this purpose, the STIPO prototype of BPO was compared to each patient's actual STIPO scores on the same variables to obtain a BPO similarity index, reflecting the similarity between the expert prototypical profile and the individual STIPO scores. This BPO similarity index was a new dimensional variable used for the following comparisons between BPO and other measures of personality disorder (hypotheses 3 to 5).

Similarity index – method

The method chosen to establish the similarity index was the squared Euclidean distance – different from Trull et al. (2003) who used intraclass Q-correlations to compute the similarity of each individual to the prototype based on 30 prototypic domains. As in the present study only four domains were used for comparison between prototype and individuals, the squared Euclidean distance was preferred to account for the limited number of variables. The squared Euclidian distance provides a similarity index for each patient, which indicates the similarity of each of the sixty individuals to the four prototypical domains.

Similarity Index – Preparatory steps and variables

The similarity index was computed by matching the four prototype domain scores of each patient to the four prototypic domains. First, for several reasons, the data was modified as follows: The prototypic domains had different cut-offs, that is a rating of "3" or larger in the domains "Identity - coherence and continuity" and "Identity - Representation of others", and "4" or larger in "Object relations" and "Primitive Defenses". The scores above these cut-offs were collapsed, so that a patient's score of 3, 4 or 5 in the first or second domain was collapsed to a score of 3. In the third and fourth domain, the scores were collapsed to a score of 4 (compare table 12). This was done because the scores above the cut-offs were considered equally prototypic. For example a patient rated with a "4" is regarded as BPO-prototypic as a patient rated with a "3". Also, this step was necessary to avoid dissimilarities which were not expected from a theoretical viewpoint, that is a patient rated with a "1" (2 rating points away from the cut-off score "3"; indicating "absence of pathology") is expected to have a large dissimilarity to the prototype, but a patient rated with a "5" (also

2 points from the cut-off score "3"; indicating "very severe pathology") is regarded similar to the prototype. Thus, the similarity was computed based on the collapsed data (ranging from 1 to 3 in the first two domains, and from 1 to 4 in the last two domains).

Table 12. Prototype: Collapsed data

Prototypic domain	Ratings regarded non-prototypical	Ratings regarded prototypical	Collapsed ratings	
Identity - coherence and continuity	1, 2	3, 4, 5	3, 4, 5	→ collapsed to 3
Identity - Representation of others	1, 2	3, 4, 5	3, 4, 5	→ collapsed to 3
Object relations	1, 2, 3	4, 5	4, 5	→ collapsed to 4
Primitive Defenses	1, 2, 3	4, 5	4, 5	→ collapsed to 4

The range of ratings in each of the four prototypic domains can also be seen in figure 3 in the previous chapter. We understand that no meaningful information was lost through collapsing the data, as there are two sequential questions to be asked when looking at each patient's results: First, the decision if one of the four prototype criteria is fulfilled depends on where the score lies – above or below the respective cut-off. Second, combining the information "prototypical or not" from this score with the information from the other three scores provides important diagnostic information if the patient is more prototypical and thus, more severely disturbed or not.

Also, no differences were found when computing the similarity index with the collapsed versus the non-collapsed data: The correlations (see hypotheses 3 and 4) between the similarity index and the other data were comparable with both.

Prototypical criteria - Frequencies

Based on the frequencies of the prototype domains in the total sample (compare table 13), it can be seen how prototypical the patients are within the sample, that is how many of the four prototype criteria they fulfill. We find different groups according to the frequencies, that is patients fulfilling none (16.7%), some (50%) or all of the criteria (33.3%). We would expect patients fulfilling all of the four criteria to be very prototypically BPO, whereas patients fulfilling none of the four criteria to be not prototypically BPO. Examination of these groupings according to number of fulfilled prototypical criteria was in part reported elsewhere (Hoerz et al., 2007) and is subject of further study. Here, groupings according to similarity to the prototype will be examined more thoroughly by studying the sample through a cluster analysis and comparing these clusters (see hypothesis 1).

Table 13. Frequencies of prototypical domains (N=60)

STIPO prototype	N		N
Met any of prototype criteria	50	4 of 4 criteria	20 (33.3%)
		1 to 3 of 4 criteria	30 (50.0%)
Met no prototype criteria	10	0 of 4 criteria	10 (16.7%)

Similarity Index – Results

Based on the collapsed scores of the 5-point dimensional ratings of the prototypical domains, the squared Euclidian distance was computed as the similarity index [2]. Thus, the STIPO scores used were solely each patient's ratings of the four prototype domains "Identity - coherence", "Identity - representation of others", "Object relations" and "Primitive defenses". The similarity of each of the 60 patients to this prototype was calculated by comparing the four collapsed patient scores to the four prototypical scores. The squared Euclidian distance served as a BPO similarity index for each patient. The similarity scores across the sample ranged from 0 (very similar, i.e. an exact match to the BPO-prototype) to - 26.00 (very dissimilar, i.e. not BPO-prototypic). The average similarity index computed across the sample lay at - 4.87 (SD= 7.07).

[2] As the Euclidian distance is conceptualized as a "dissimilarity measure", the squared Euclidian distance was multiplied with (-1) to yield a "similarity index". Computations based on this "similarity index" will be presented for ease of reading.

Table 14. Similarity index across the sample

	M	SD	Min	Max
Similarity index based on four prototypical domains	- 4.87	7.07	0	- 26.00

M = mean, *SD* = standard deviation, *Min* = Minimum, *Max* = Maximum

Clusters according to similarity to the prototype

After the similarity index, which indicates the similarity of each individual to the prototype, had been computed, another question was investigated: How do clusters which emerge according to the similarity index differ from one another? Can the four variables that form the prototype of BPO be used to create clinically meaningful and distinct groups of patients? In order to examine these questions, a hierarchical cluster analysis was computed with the four prototypical domains entered as first case and the 60 patients' domain scores. Several efforts were done to find the best cluster solution. These clusters and their properties on external variables will then be examined more in detail in section 1.4.

The graphic presentation of the results from the cluster analysis is the dendrogram (figure 4), the aggregation of the 60 patients into different clusters according to their similarity to the prototype. The clusters are as internally homogeneous as possible (i.e. minimum within sum of squares) and the various clusters are as different as possible from each other. The dendrogram shows which cases were joined together into clusters and at what distance, and at later stages, which clusters were joined together into larger clusters, and at what distance. The distance is shown on the vertical axis as the "rescaled distance cluster combine", which is the increase of heterogeneity when more clusters are combined. The scale which presents this has a range from 0 to 25 and is a normed version of the fusion coefficient from the agglomeration process.
Horizontally, the cases represent the 60 patients. In the dendrogram, the graphic representation shows that a useful solution is a three-cluster solution, taking a rescaled distance of 8 as the cut-off for an acceptable level of the heterogeneity measure (Backhaus et al., 2003). Also, the three-cluster solution was confirmed in the agglomeration schedule by the jump in the distance coefficient at the

transition from the 4-cluster to the 3-cluster solution. The three major clusters differed according to their similarity to the prototype (operationalized by the distance d from the prototype). The largest group has 43 subjects (cluster 1; d= 0 to -6), cluster 2 consists of 10 subjects (d= -5 to -13) and cluster 3 has 7 patients (d= -17 to -26). The additional division into clusters 1a, 1b, 1c is for descriptive purposes only and did not undergo any group statistical analyses. In the section describing the single cases these subgroups are taken into consideration.

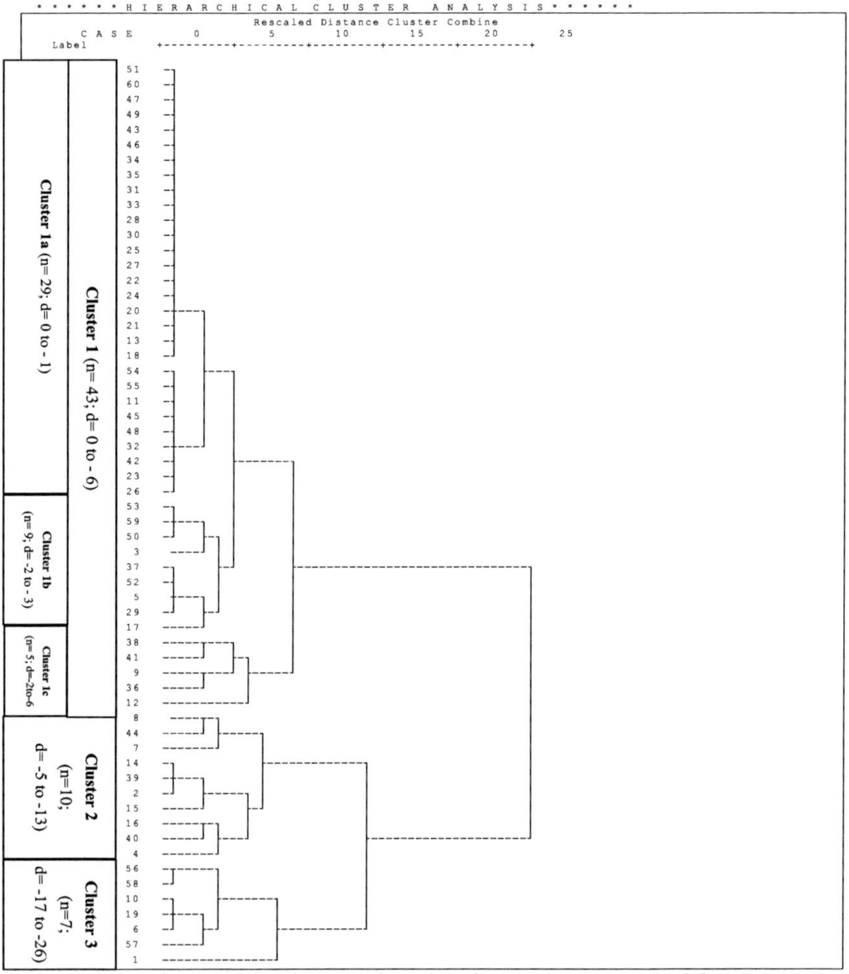

Figure 4. Dendrogram from cluster analysis, based on the four prototypical domains

In order to test this three-cluster cluster solution and to see if the distribution of the patients into these clusters could be replicated and is of use, two additional cluster analyses were computed. First, a k-means cluster analysis was calculated with the data, choosing a 3-cluster solution. The resulting clusters are roughly of similar size, the first cluster including 33 patients, the second cluster 17 patients and the third cluster ten patients. The majority of patients were still part of the same clusters in both procedures. The patients who were "moved" from the first group of the hierarchical cluster analysis to the second group (i.e. 10 patients) when computing the k-means procedure were patients who were assigned rather high d-scores in the hierarchical analysis, that is patients who were less similar to the prototype.
Also, to test if the three cluster solution as found with the hierarchical cluster analysis was correct and to examine if the same groups were found when a different method for the cut-off-score (i.e. the score on the 5-point scale of the prototypical domains determining prototypicality), another cluster analysis was computed. For this, the data above and below the cut-off score on the 1-5 point scale was modified as follows: The data was changed to "prototypical- yes or no" in each of the four domains and then a cluster analysis was computed with these dichotomized scores. The scores in each of the four domains were changed to dichotomous scores, that is scores below the cut-off score were coded as a "0", whereas scores above the cut-off scores were coded as a "1". For example, in the domain "coherence and continuity", ratings of "1" and "2" were recoded to "0" and ratings of "3 through 5" were recoded to "1". With these dichotomous ratings, for each patient the similarity to the prototype was computed with a hierarchical cluster analysis. The clusters evolving from this procedure again were roughly comparable to the results from the previous analyses: The largest cluster consisted of 31 patients, the second of 18 patients and the third of 11 patients. Given the fact that in the three different cluster procedures clusters of roughly comparable size and composition were found, the cut-off-point for the similarity index and the cluster solution based on it were considered to be confirmed and to be analyzed further.

The clusters present patient groups aggregated according to closeness to the four prototypical domains. The clusters differ as to how many of the prototypical criteria the patients fulfill and how close their ratings are to the BPO prototype, that is how severe the borderline pathology is. Below, figure 5 shows the sample divided into the clusters according closeness to the prototype. It clearly can be seen that in the first cluster the highest number of prototype criteria were fulfilled; on average three criteria, followed by cluster 2 in which on average one criterion was fulfilled. In cluster 3, only one patient fulfilled one of the criteria, the remaining patients fulfilled none of the criteria. The next questions to be examined are if these groups are different on external variables and which of the prototype criteria are fulfilled in the respective clusters. These questions will be studied in the chapter "Hypothesis 1".

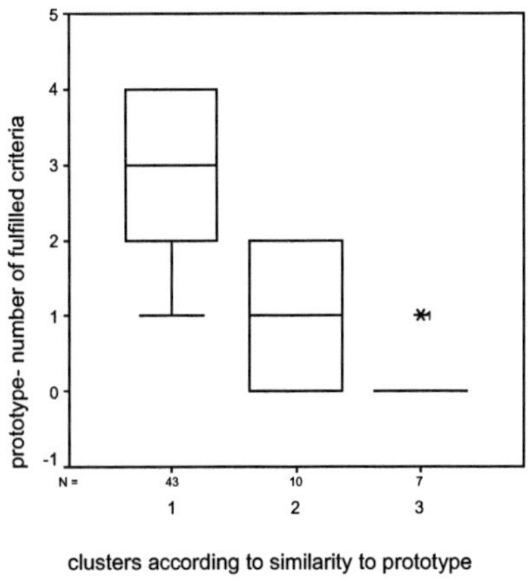

Figure 5. Number of fulfilled prototypical criteria across the clusters

1.4. Hypothesis 1: Clinical groups according to BPO prototype

According to the first hypothesis, we expect the BPO prototype to discriminate between clinically relevant groups in our sample of patients, different in general pathology, levels of axis I and axis II pathology. For this question the clusters which had been formed by the cluster analysis in the previous section will be examined more in detail. These clusters which had emerged by entering the dimensional ratings of the four prototypical domains of each patient into the cluster analysis will be scrutinized in two steps: first, the distribution of prototypical criteria across the clusters will be inspected, then they will be compared by means of a one-way analysis of variance (ANOVA) in order to see if they are meaningfully different from each other on external variables.

1.4.1 Prototype criteria across the clusters

The distribution of the four prototypical domains across and within the three clusters will be examined. Figures 6 to 9 show the four prototype domains across the clusters, with the two bars showing if the respective prototype had been fulfilled (dark bar) or not (light bar).

Cluster 1 – the BPO cluster

All of the patients fulfilled prototypical criteria, 46.5% fulfilled all four, 53.5% fulfilled between one and three criteria. The most frequent criterion in which patients from this cluster reached the prototypical score was "representation of others" (93%), followed by "coherence" (88%) and "primitive defenses" (74.4%). The criterion the least of the patients fulfilled was "object relations" (55.8%).

Cluster 2 – the intermediate cluster

In cluster 2, four of the ten patients met no prototypical criteria and six patients met between one and three criteria. None met all of the criteria. Thus, this cluster can be considered not as prototypical as the first. When examining where the focus lay, i.e. which of the criteria were fulfilled most frequently, it is very clear that the difficulties with "representation of others" was predominant in this group (60% reached the prototypical score). Only 30% were prototypical in "coherence and continuity", 10% in "object relations" and none of the patients (0%) reached the cut-off for the BPO-prototype in "primitive defenses". Thus, this intermediate group presents the most difficulties with perceiving others and being sensible for social cues and realities. One might wonder why four of the patients met none of the prototype criteria and still were assigned to this cluster. These patients were below the cut-off for prototypicality in the four domains, but were *close* to it, showing some similarity to the prototype. For example, some of them reached a score of 3 in the domain "primitive defenses", which clearly indicates some use of primitive defenses but does not imply serious impairment in daily functioning due to this defense style. Hence, they might be considered higher level BPO patients. According to the distribution of the BPO prototype criteria, this cluster will be called an intermediate group.

Cluster 3 – the NPO cluster

In the third cluster, only one of the patients met one of the prototypical criteria. This patient reached a score of "3" in the domain "representation of others". The other patients had no scores above the cut-off for the BPO prototype in any of the domains.

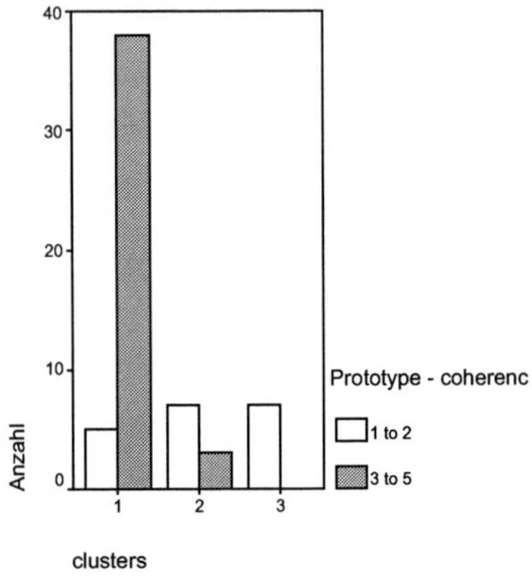

Figure 6. Prototype criterion 1: "Coherence and continuity" across the three clusters (1 to 2 = not prototypical, 3 to 5 = prototypical)

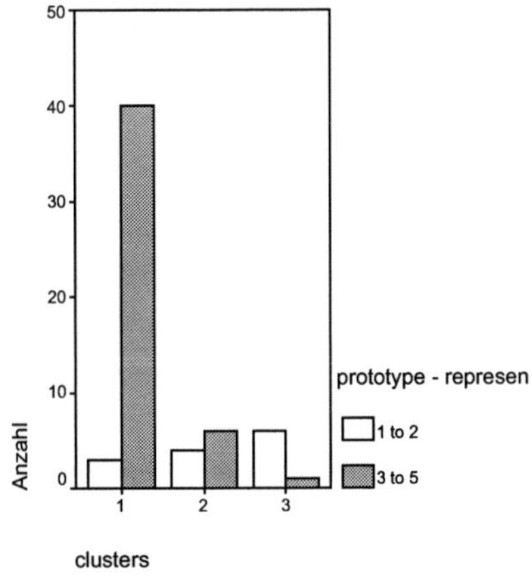

Figure 7. Prototype criterion 2: "Representations of others" across the three clusters (1 to 2 = not prototypical, 3 to 5= prototypical)

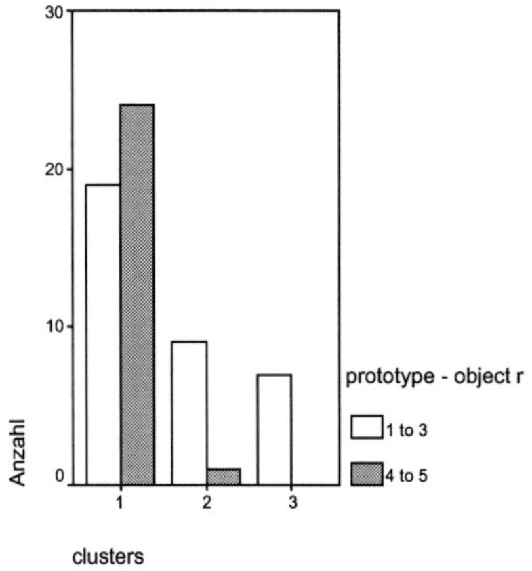

Figure 8. Prototype criterion 3: "Object relations" across the three clusters (1 to 3 = not prototypical, 4to 5= prototypical)

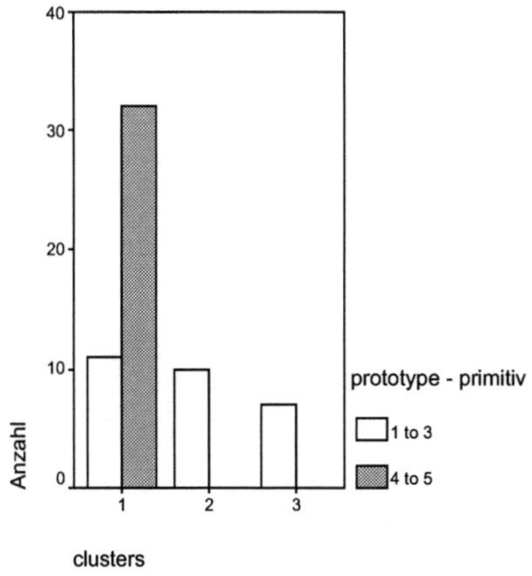

Figure 9. Prototype criterion 4: "Primitive defenses" across the three clusters (1 to 3 = not prototypical, 4 to 5= prototypical)

Summarizing the results regarding the prototype criteria across the three clusters, one can state that the predominant area the patients had difficulties with was "representation of others", indicating that this might be the most sensitive domain of the four prototypical domains. Compare figure 10 for this, which shows the relative frequency of each of the four prototypical domains across the three clusters. The bars indicate the amount of patients (in %) per cluster who fulfilled the prototype.

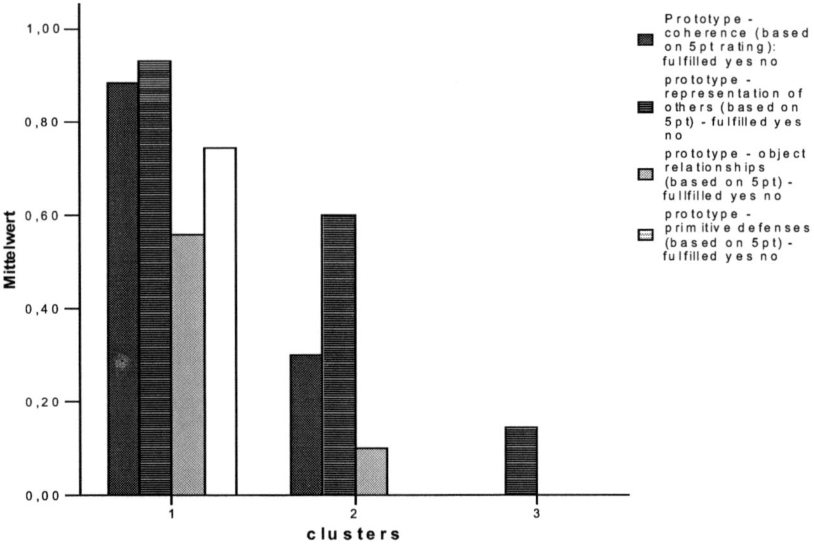

Figure 10. Proportion of the four prototype criteria across clusters

As an example, in the first cluster, 88% of the patients fulfilled the prototype in the domain "coherence", i.e. reached a score equal or higher than 3. In the domain "representation of others", 93% were above the cut-off, whereas in the domain "object relations", 56% were above the cutoff in this domain, and lastly, 74% were in the prototypical range of the domain "primitive defenses". For the interpretation of these results, it is of importance to note that in the construction of the prototype, the "cut-off" for the prototypical range was higher, i.e. more specific in the domains "object relations" and "primitive defenses". This means that lower numbers of fulfilled criteria in these two prototype domains (across all three clusters) might be explained through these higher cutoffs. Again, it is of high interest that in all three of the clusters, the domain "representation of others" was the most pathological of the four prototypical domains. In cluster 1, 93% of the patients were above the cutoff, in the second cluster 60% of the patients were in the prototypical range, and even in the healthiest cluster 3, one of the patients (14%) was in the prototypical range of this domain, rated with a 3.

Overall, the distribution of the prototype criteria across the clusters and across the sample is as expected, that is the most and highest pathology in cluster 1, clearly less in cluster 2 and nearly no pathology in cluster 3. The mean scores (on the clinical 5-point ratings) of the four domains in cluster 1 were 3.8 in coherence, 3.9 in representation of others, 3.6 in object relations and 4.0 in primitive defenses. In cluster 2 the respective means were 2.3, 2.9, 2.7 and 1.7. Finally, in the third cluster the mean scores were 1.0, 1.6., 1.6 and 1.0.

1.4.2 Comparison of clusters on external measures

According to the first hypothesis, we expect the BPO prototype to discriminate between relevant clinical groups in our sample of patients, showing differences in general pathology, levels of axis I and axis II pathology. The three groups, emerged from the cluster analysis, were examined with a one-way ANOVA in order to see if they were meaningfully different from each other.

The interest in the results from this procedure is two-fold. One is to examine if the grouping the cluster analysis came up with is useful. A cluster analysis is a method which always produces a grouping, but these may or may not prove useful for grouping subjects with similar features. Thus, it is an important step to see if the clusters are different on variables not used to do the grouping. This significance test on external variables is one of the best validation techniques for cluster analyses according to Aldenderfer and Blashfield (1984, p.66). Second, the major goal of this study is to examine the usefulness of the BPO prototype based on the STIPO interview. If the grouping provides sensible clusters we find confirmation both for the method and for the instrument itself.

The three groups from the dendrogramm (figure 4) were examined with a one-way analysis of variance regarding differences on external variables. Several measures were taken into consideration as outcome variables: To evaluate general pathology, the General Assessment of Functioning score (GAF; from DSM-IV (APA; 1994) assessed by clinicians independent from the study), and the general severity index from the self report “Brief Symptom Inventory” were examined. Albeit not an external instrument, the differentiation through the similarity index in the STIPO domain “Coping and Rigidity” (which was not part of the prototype) was considered as well hypothesizing that coping skills might diverge according to cluster membership as well. This domain was also

considered an index of general functioning. To assess axis I pathology, the BSI subscales were considered and to inspect the clusters for differences in axis II pathology, the SNAP diagnostic scales. In addition to this, some scales from the aforementioned self report instruments, that is SNAP temperament scales, IIP-PD, IPO, PANAS, Buss-Durkee Scale, and STIPO Aggression scales were examined to inspect the kind of subgroups that had emerged.
Of course, the results concerning the different clusters have to be interpreted carefully as the number of subjects per cluster deviates quite a bit and generalizations cannot be made easily. To account for the different sample sizes, levene tests on homogeneity of variances were conducted. In the case of heterogenic variances ($p < .05$), the Welch Statistic was conducted and the appropriate post-hoc tests were chosen (Games-Howell). If variances were homogenous, ANOVA F-tests and Tukey post-hoc tests were conducted. Both post hoc tests took into account the cumulated alpha error (Bonferroni correction). All variables were tested with regard to normal distribution (Kolmogorov-Smirnov-Test; $p < .05$). For non-normally distributed variables, the results were additionally tested with nonparametric procedures (Kruskal-Wallis-H-Test) and as the results remained on the same levels of significance, they were considered to be confirmed. An alpha level of .05 was used for all statistical tests. The means and standard deviations as well as the Welch and F-statistic and levels of significance resulting from the one-way ANOVAs are displayed in tables 15 through 17, separated into a) general pathology, b) axis I symptoms and c) axis II symptoms and correlates.

General pathology across the clusters

Examining the clusters according to general functioning (GAF score from DSM-IV, APA, 1994) and the GSI (General Severity Index from the BSI), it is apparent that significant differences exist between the first, largest cluster and both of the other clusters. Regarding the GAF Scores, cluster differences could be found. As the levene test on homogenous variances had proven significant, the Welch Statistic was computed, resulting in a significant score (44.17, $p < .001$). Follow-up Games-Howell post hoc tests showed that the paired-group differences lay between groups 1 and 2 ($p < .05$) as well as 1 and 3 ($p < .001$). Similar results were obtained for the GSI (see figure 11), indicating that the first cluster shows significantly more pathology and deficits in general functioning than the second and third cluster. The boxplots also illustrate that the second and third cluster are not significantly different from each other and thus can be considered not as disturbed as the first group of patients. Finally, conceptualizing an individual's coping skills as an index of general functioning, the STIPO subdomain "Coping and Rigidity" was also analyzed with a oneway ANOVA. It showed significant differences between the clusters (F (2,57)= 30.47; $p < .001$) and Tukey post-hoc pairwise comparisons demonstrated significant differences between clusters 1 and 2 ($p < .001$) and between clusters 1 and 3 ($p < .001$).

Table 15. Differences in means across the different BPO-prototype based clusters: a) general pathology (N= 60)

	Cluster 1 (n= 43)		Cluster 2 (n=10)		Cluster 3 (n=7)					
	M	*SD*	*M*	*SD*	*M*	*SD*	*levene*	*F (2, 57)*	*Welch*	*Post-hoc*
GAF	43.64	16.12	64.38	15.91	77.50	5.24	.04		**44.17*****	1-2* 1-3***
BSI GSI	1.69	.77	.70	.74	.33	.26	.09	**15.42*****		1-2** 1-3***
STIPO Coping/ Rigidity	4.26	.79	2.90	.74	2.00	1.00	.25	**30.47*****		1-2*** 1-3***

* $p < .05$; ** $p < .01$; *** $p < .001$; *N/S*: not significant; M = mean, SD = standard deviation
GAF = General Assessment of Functioning (SCID Interview). Note that higher SCID GAF scores indicate better functioning; BSI GSI = BSI General Severity Index

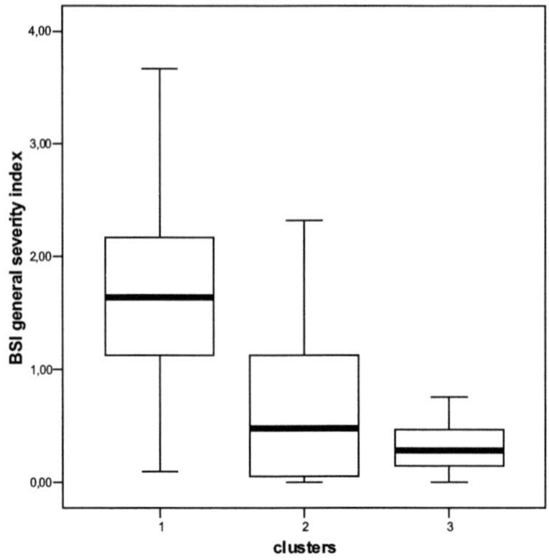

Figure 11. Boxplots of clusters: BSI GSI scale

Axis I pathology across the clusters

Further, the clusters were analyzed according to levels of axis I pathology, taking the BSI subscales as indices of several axis I disorders, for example phobic anxiety being closely related to anxiety disorders. In table 16 it is shown that on all BSI subscales, significant differences were found between the three clusters, primarily between the first cluster as it compares to the second and third.

For example, the one way analysis of variance indicated a significant effect of cluster membership in the scale "obsessive-compulsiveness" ($F(2, 57) = 12.10$, $p < .001$). Post hoc Tukey's tests demonstrated that the significant difference arose between clusters 1 and 2 ($p < .05$) as well as 1 and 3 ($p < .001$). Again, in most of the comparisons it becomes clear that clusters 2 and 3 seem to be more similar (i.e. less pathological) than cluster 1 (more pathological).

Table 16. Differences in means across the different BPO-prototype based clusters: b) axis I pathology assessed by BSI subscales (N= 60)

	Cluster 1 (n= 43)		Cluster 2 (n=10)		Cluster 3 (n=7)					
	M	*SD*	*M*	*SD*	*M*	*SD*	*levene*	*F (2, 57)*	*Welch*	*Post-hoc*
Somatization	.92	.76	.36	.60	.08	.11	.05	**6.12****		1-3**
Obsessive-compulsive	1.98	.93	.95	.92	.48	.49	.19	**12.10*****		1-2* 1-3***
Interpersonal sensitivity	2.42	1.09	.93	1.08	.71	.68	.26	**13.84*****		1-2*** 1-3***
Depression	2.43	1.17	1.08	1.31	.64	.57	.04		**20.62*****	1-2* 1-3***
Anxiety	1.73	.95	.92	1.13	.38	.31	.04		**25.14*****	1-2* 1-3**
Hostility	1.41	1.12	.44	.58	.29	.30	.00		**15.06*****	1-2** 1-3***
Phobic anxiety	1.32	1.00	.34	.54	.03	.08	.00		**35.10*****	1-2*** 1-3***
Paranoid ideation	1.44	1.02	.52	.79	.20	.35	.02		**18.26*****	1-2* 1-3***
Psychoticism	1.68	.93	.70	.88	.17	.18	.04		**45.09*****	1-2* 1-3***

* $p < .05$; ** $p < .01$; *** $p < .001$; *N/S*: not significant; *M* = mean, *SD* = standard deviation
Note: All scales are BSI subscales.

Figure 12 shows the differences across the clusters in the subdomain "Phobic anxiety"; the highest amount of pathology was found in cluster 1. The sole BSI subdomain in which significant differences could be found only between clusters 1 and 3 is "somatization". In this case, the second cluster shows more pathology, indicating the degree of somatization of this patient group leaning towards that of the first cluster.

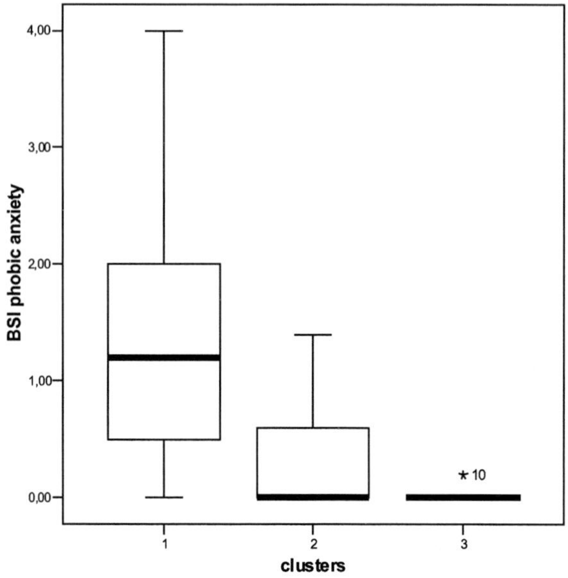

Figure 12. Boxplots of clusters: BSI phobic anxiety scale

Axis II pathology across the clusters

Another important aspect was how the clusters differed according to axis II pathology and domains associated with axis II, for example the diagnostic scales from the SNAP or important indices of axis II pathology like the IIP-PD. Also, to answer the question if the clusters diverged regarding the structural level, the analysis was conducted with the IPO scales as well. Table 17 shows that in all of the comparisons between the three clusters, significant differences could be found, with the exception of the SNAP histrionic personality disorder scale and the IPO Reality Testing scale. In the majority of cases, the pattern found in the first two analyses (general functioning, axis I) was replicated: The first cluster was significantly more impaired than the second and the third cluster.

Table 17. Differences in means across the different BPO-prototype based clusters: c) measures of axis II pathology (N= 60)

		Cluster 1 (n= 43)		Cluster 2 (n=10)		Cluster 3 (n=7)					
		M	*SD*	*M*	*SD*	*M*	*SD*	*levene*	*F (2, 57)*	*Welch*	*Post-hoc*
	Par	11.79	6.08	5.40	5.68	3.00	2.77	.02		**19.84*****	1-2* 1-3***
	Schiz	7.26	3.56	3.50	3.10	3.29	1.60	.02		**13.16*****	1-2** 1-3***
	Schiz.typ	10.47	4.85	5.70	4.30	3.14	2.27	.09	**10.58*****		1-2** 1-3***
	Antisoc	10.72	5.43	6.30	3.80	3.86	3.53	.21	**7.58****		1-2* 1-3**
	BPD	15.93	5.22	8.20	5.43	4.43	2.44	.26	**21.88*****		1-2*** 1-3***
	Narc.	8.63	4.25	6.10	2.69	4.43	2.51	.06	**4.55***		1-3*
	Histr.	8.72	3.71	9.70	4.76	7.71	2.81	.38	**.57**		N/S
	Av.	12.05	4.28	7.40	4.35	4.86	2.54	.46	**12.30*****		1-2** 1-3***
	Dep.	11.77	5.14	7.50	4.38	3.29	3.73	.17	**10.69*****		1-2* 1-3***
SNAP	Obc.	12.81	3.32	10.50	3.47	9.14	3.80	.67	**4.68***		1-3*
	Neg temp	22.40	5.75	14.20	8.35	7.57	7.41	.10	**19.85*****		1-2** 1-3***
	Mistrust	12.05	3.39	5.90	4.15	1.43	.53	.02		**17.46*****	1-3***
	Manip	1.72	.81	.92	.73	.69	.40	.07	**9.06*****		1-2** 1-3**
	Aggr	2.97	.74	2.20	.57	1.90	.59	.01		**18.60*****	1-2* 1-3***
	Selfharm	2.75	.74	2.13	.47	1.50	.36	.01		**176.76*****	1-2** 1-3*** 2-3*
	SH – low self esteem	5.76	1.56	2.70	1.95	.43	0.53	.06	**44.87*****		1-2*** 1-3*** 2-3*
	SH – suicide proneness	6.43	2.53	3.2	2.66	.57	.79	.05		**19.82*****	1-2** 1-3*** 2-3*
	SNAP Impulsivity	8.88	4.33	5.6	2.99	4.29	3.77	.25	**5.55****		1-3*

	IIP-PD	1.72	.81	.92	.73	.69	.40	.25	**8.51****		1-2** 1-3**
	IPO Identity	2.97	.74	2.20	.57	1.90	.59	.40	**10.31*****		1-2** 1-3**
	IPO Primitive Defenses	2.75	.74	2.13	.47	1.50	.36	.08	**12.31*****		1-2* 1-3***
I P O	IPO Aggression	2.02	.70	1.26	.26	1.22	.24	.05	**9.67*****		1-2** 1-3**
	IPO Moral Values	2.34	.61	1.63	.39	1.52	.66	.11	**10.14*****		1-2** 1-3**
	IPO Real. Test.	1.87	.60	1.43	.37	1.36	.27	.17	**4.53***		N/S
	PANAS pos. aff.	22.93	8.16	30.20	7.98	31.00	9.11	.68	**5.20****		1-2*
	PANAS neg. aff.	31.93	9.17	21.30	7.78	14.14	3.63	.05	**16.05*****		1-2** 1-3***
	Buss-Durk. Irritability	7.23	2.77	4.30	3.27	3.29	2.14	.50	**9.02*****		1-2** 1-3**
	STIPO self-directed aggress.	4.02	1.28	2.50	1.80	1.14	.38	.00		**19.57*****	1-3***
	STIPO other-directed aggress.	2.91	1.27	1.30	.67	1.29	.49	.01		**20.13*****	1-2*** 1-3***

* $p < .05$; ** $p < .01$; *** $p < .001$; *N/S*: not significant; M = mean, SD = standard deviation

Axis II symptoms

As an example for the dimensional scores on the SNAP diagnostic scales, the one way analysis indicated a significant effect of cluster membership on the SNAP borderline personality disorder dimensional score ($F(2, 57) = 21.88$, $p < .001$). Post hoc Tukey's tests documented statistically significant differences between clusters 1 and 2 as well as 1 and 3 ($p < .001$). In the other SNAP diagnostic scales, similar results were found: the dimensional scores were higher in cluster 1 than in clusters 2 or 3. Interestingly, only the scores of narcissistic personality disorder and obsessive-compulsive personality disorder, no significant difference was found between clusters 1 and 2. This might indicate that cluster 2 is more similar to the first cluster in narcissism and obsessive traits. In figure 13, as example for the SNAP personality disorders, the boxplots based on the BPD dimensional ratings are shown. The median of the dimensional BPD score in cluster 1 is 16, whereas in cluster 2 it is 8.5 and in cluster 3 it is 4.

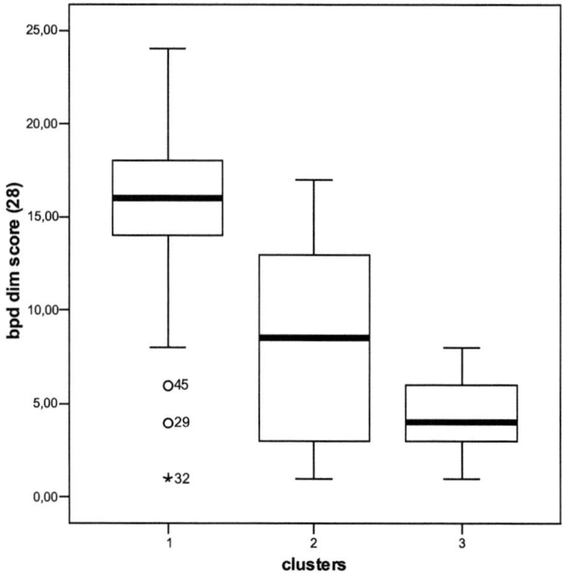

Figure 13. Boxplots of clusters: SNAP BPD scale

Also, the distribution of the different SNAP personality disorders across the clusters is of interest. One question is if there are differences in the distribution of higher level and lower level personality diagnoses when comparing the three clusters. The frequencies of SNAP personality disorders were computed with the SNAP categorical personality disorder diagnoses, in contrast to the dimensional scores used in the analyses of variance when comparing the clusters previously. Based on the categorical diagnoses, most patients in cluster 1 are assigned at least one personality disorder (81.4%) and the average number of SNAP personality disorders per patient is 1.9. In cluster 2, only 50% of the patients are assigned a SNAP personality disorder, and the average number of personality disorders is 0.6. In cluster 3 no SNAP personality disorder diagnosis is met.

Thus, the number of diagnoses matches the decrease of pathology from cluster 1 through 3 found so far.

But does cluster 1 include more lower level, more disturbed personality disorders than cluster 2? Following Kernberg's classification of personality disorders, which for example regards antisocial personality disorder as the most disturbed and obsessive-compulsive personality disorder as one of the higher level personality disorders (compare figure 1), a specific distribution of personality disorders across the clusters is expected; lower level personality disorders in the first group of patients, higher level personality disorders in the second group of patients. A rather varied distribution of personality disorders in the two clusters is found, shown in table 18. In fact, in cluster 1, the majority of patients does obtain one or more of the higher level personality disorder diagnoses like avoidant personality disorder (54%), followed by dependent personality disorder (33%), while lower level personality disorders like borderline personality disorder (33%), antisocial (9%), schizoid (9%), schizotypal (12%) or paranoid (19%) were assigned as well. In cluster 2, the most frequent personality disorder diagnosis was histrionic personality disorder (20%), followed by avoidant (10%), dependent (10%), borderline (10%), and paranoid personality disorder (10%). Note that many patients were assigned several personality disorders. Comparing both clusters, the frequencies indicate that while the severely disturbed personality disorders like antisocial or schizoid personality disorder were found in the first and most disturbed cluster, they were not assigned in cluster 2.

An interesting finding is that the amount of histrionic personality disorders was twice as high in the "intermediate" cluster than in the first cluster. These findings are in line with Kernberg's classification. Somewhat surprising, but in line with findings on co-occurrence of personality disorders, the so-called higher level personality disorders like avoidant or dependent personality disorders were present in both clusters.

Due to the fact that multiple diagnoses could be assigned per patient (some patients received up to four diagnoses), the interpretation of these findings is complicated. For example, one might presume that if the diagnoses had been given by a clinician, some would be regarded primary, others secondary diagnoses. As these results rely on self-report data, no such distinction can be made.

Table 18. Frequencies of patients meeting criteria for SNAP personality disorder, across the three BPO-based clusters (N= 60)

	Cluster 1 (n=43)	Cluster 2 (n=10)	Cluster 3 (n=7)
Paranoid PD	19%	10%	0%
Schizoid PD	9%	0%	0%
Schizotypal PD	12%	0%	0%
Antisocial PD	9%	0%	0%
Borderline PD	33%	10%	0%
Narcissistic PD	7%	0%	0%
Histrionic PD	9%	20%	0%
Avoidant PD	54%	10%	0%
Dependent PD	33%	10%	0%
Obsessive-Compulsive PD	19%	0%	0%

Note: based on SNAP categorical scoring method; several diagnoses per patient could be assigned

Axis II correlates across the clusters

Also in the SNAP temperament scales, the PANAS "Negative Affect", and the Buss-Durkee "Irritability" scale, significant differences were found between the groups (see table for F-scores). In the SNAP Scales "Negative Temperament", "Manipulativeness", and "Aggression" were significantly higher in cluster 1 than in clusters 2 and 3, as was shown through significant post hoc pairwise comparisons.

Similarly, clusters 2 and 3 showed a lot of similarity on the other variables of axis II pathology. For example, in the IIP-PD mean score, an important index measuring functional impairment in the interpersonal domain, no significant results were found between these clusters. Figure 14 shows that significant differences between the clusters could be found ($F(2, 57) = 8.51, p < .01$), both between clusters 1 and 2 as well as between 1 and 3 ($p < .01$). The medians of clusters 2 and 3 are identical, although the second cluster comprises a broader range of IIP-PD scores.

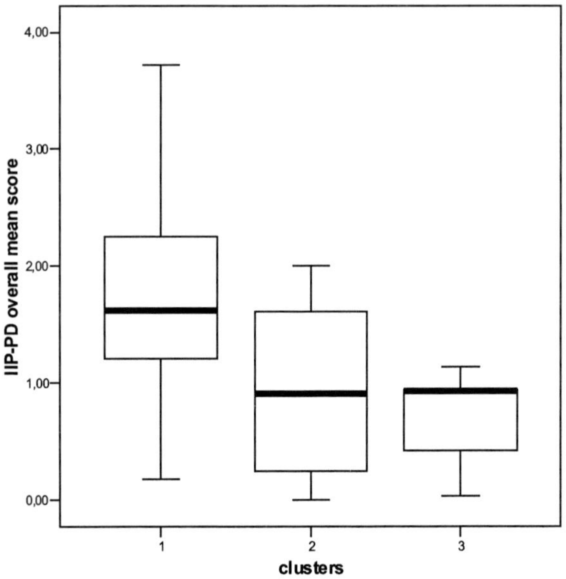

Figure 14. Boxplots of clusters: IIP-PD scale

Furthermore, in order to examine if the clusters which resulted from the analysis according to the BPO prototype showed differences in personality organization or structure, the IPO Identity and Primitive Defenses scales were examined as to how different these scales were across the clusters. These IPO domains are regarded as key elements in borderline pathology and are expected to discriminate between BPO and NPO. On the one hand, the IPO domains have similar content as the STIPO domains (which are the basis for the BPO prototype), but as the IPO is an independent self-report measure it can be regarded as an external measure compared to the STIPO. Moreover, the results in the IPO in this section are very important for the construct validity of these key domains of BPO. If convergent results are found across different assessment modes (i.e. self-report IPO and interview STIPO), this strongly contributes to the construct validity of these BPO key domains identity or primitive defenses. The degree of overlap between STIPO and IPO will be further examined in hypothesis 5.

In the IPO domain "Identity", significant differences between the clusters were found (F (2, 57) = 10.31, $p < .001$). Post hoc Tukey comparisons documented statistically significant differences between clusters 1 and 2 ($p < .01$) and between clusters 1 and 3 ($p < .001$). Similarly, in the domain "Primitive Defenses", clusters 1 and 2 were different ($p < .05$) as well as clusters 1 and 3 ($p < .001$). Figure 15 presents the results from this domain in a boxplot. Thus, the convergent finding of STIPO-based and IPO-based pathology in the domain "primitive defenses" can be regarded an important result with regard to the construct validity of this concept.

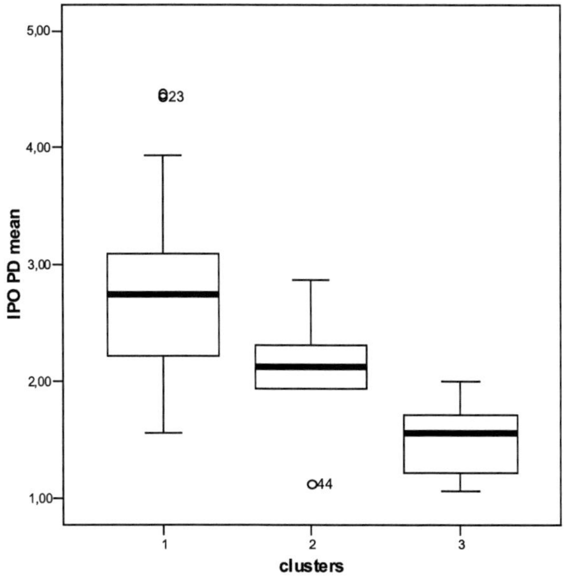

Figure 15. Boxplots of clusters: IPO Primitive Defenses scale

Measures of self harm across the clusters

Interestingly, in the SNAP scale "self-harm", differences between all three groups were found (compare table 17). As the levene test on homogenous variances had proven significant, the Welch Statistic was computed, resulting in a significant score (176,76***, $p < .001$). Follow-up Games-Howell post hoc tests showed that the paired-group differences lay between groups 1 and 2 ($p <$

.01), 2 and 3 ($p < .05$) and between 1 and 3 ($p < .001$). The observed difference between the second and third cluster was not found in any of the other scales, suggesting that this might be a domain which discriminates between the clusters very well. Figure 16 shows this variable in boxplots. Even when examining the two subscales of this SNAP domain, "selfharm – low self-esteem" and "selfharm – suicide proneness", the significant differences remained between all three clusters, indicating a meaningful difference between the three groups with respect to self-harming thoughts as well as behaviors (see table 17 for test statistics).

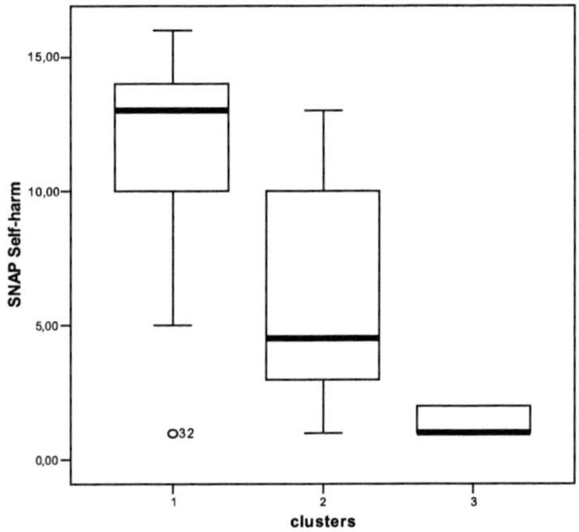

Figure 16. Boxplots of clusters: SNAP selfharm scale

Following up on these results concerning self-directed aggression, two additional variables which had been assessed by chart review of the majority of patients, were examined: History of self- injury and history of suicidal behavior had been assessed in a dichotomous format (yes - no). Unfortunately, due to missing data, only 30 patients from the first cluster, eight patients from the second and six patients from the first cluster could be examined. Interesting results were found which of course have to be interpreted with caution due to the smaller sample sizes. Inspecting the frequencies (compare figure 17), in the first cluster 60% of the patients report self-injurious behavior and 63% report a history of suicide attempt. In the second cluster, 13% report self-injuring behavior and 38% have a history of suicidal behavior. In cluster 3, none of the patients has a history of self-injury or suicide. In a Chi-Square-Test, significant differences between the groups were found with regard to "history of self-injury" ($\chi 2$= 11.09; $p < .01$) and with regard to "history of suicide attempt" ($\chi 2$= 8.50; $p < .05$). In order to examine the group differences post-hoc, additional Fisher exact tests were computed for each of the cluster comparisons. Significant differences between clusters 1 and 2 were found regarding history of self-injury (Fischer exact test, $p < .05$) but not regarding history of suicide attempts (Fisher exact test, $p = .19$). Compared to cluster 3, more patients in cluster 1 reported both a history of self-injury (Fisher exact test, $p < .01$) and of suicide attempts (Fisher exact test, $p < .01$). No significant differences were found between cluster 2 and 3 regarding self-injuries (Fisher exact test, $p = .57$) or regarding suicide attempts (Fisher exact test, $p = .15$). These results indicate that several patients in cluster 2 have a history of suicide attempts which moves this group closer to cluster 1 with respect to this variable. Clusters 2 and 3 again show no statistically significant difference in this comparison which stands in contrast to the results from the SNAP selfharm scale.

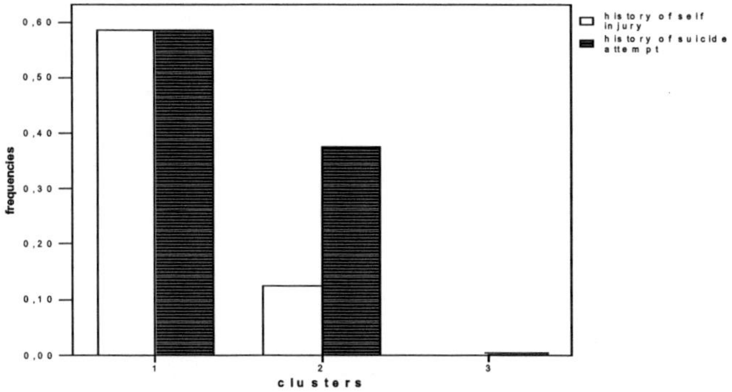

Figure 17. History of self injury and of suicide attempts across the clusters

Further, the STIPO domains "self-directed aggression" and "other-directed aggression" were analyzed (see table 17 for results). Albeit not an external instrument, these scales were included as they were not part of the prototype and because special interest was put on the question of selfharming behaviors which are assessed by a separate section in the STIPO. The mean scores of the three clusters in both of these domains were examined. As the levene test on homogenous variances had proven significant, the Welch Statistic was computed to test significant differences between the clusters, resulting in a significant score (19.57***, $p < .001$). Follow-up Games-Howell post hoc tests showed that the paired-group differences lay only between groups 1 and 3 ($p < .001$). Interestingly, on the scales “self-directed aggression”, similarly to the question of history of suicides, no difference between cluster 1 and 2 could be found, indicating these two groups’ similarity on this variable. Regarding other-directed aggression, cluster 1 was significantly different from clusters 2 and 3.

Summarizing the differences between the three clusters in a) general functioning, b) axis I pathology and c) axis II pathology, a clear pattern can be found: First, regarding the distribution of the prototypic across the clusters, it was shown (compare figure 18) that the majority of patients who fulfilled prototypical criteria were found in clusters 1 and 2, but also one patient fulfilling one of the criteria was in cluster 3 (the NPO cluster). The first cluster evidently shows the most pathology, confirmed by statistically significant differences from the other two clusters. Clusters 2 and 3 show some differences in pathology, albeit not statistically significant in the analysis of variance procedures. Translating this into clinical groups, it seems that the first group is the most disturbed, both in axis I and II symptoms and has the lowest ability to cope with its difficulties (e.g. STIPO coping skills averaging at 4.26 on a scale ranging from 1 to 5; GAF mean score of 43.64, scale ranging from 1 to 100). The second group seems to be an intermediate group, not as disturbed as the first, but still on a lower level of health (exemplified by an average GAF score of 65) than the third group. The latter is the group which seems to function the best (e.g. a mean GAF score of 77.50). Also on scales of personality pathology, the differences between the groups could be replicated, showing significant differences between group 1 and 2, and 1 and 3. The only domain in which all three groups are different from each other is the SNAP domain “selfharm”, implying that this scale (as well as the two subscales “low self-esteem” and “suicide proneness”) might be a good discriminator between our clinical groups. Importantly, when assessing self-directed aggression and suicidality by chart review, or by the STIPO self-directed aggression domain, cluster 1 and 2 are not significantly different, implying that this is an important area when inspecting the second cluster’s pathology.

As a consequence of these analyses, one might ask if groups 2 and 3 should be separate or combined. In spite of the lack of significant differences in most of the post-hoc pairwise comparisons between these clusters, this division might be of relevance for clinical reasons. A group located between severe pathology and health must be diagnosed with more care and adequate treatment must be considered carefully.

Along with these thoughts, the structural diagnosis should be given utmost priority, considering different treatments for BPO and NPO patients. As an example, it seems important to provide a patient who is closer to BPO than to NPO with a treatment focusing on structural deficits.

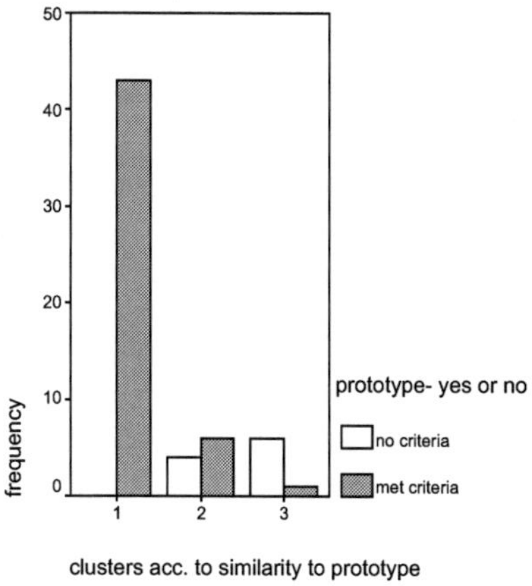

Figure 18. Distribution of prototype criteria across the clusters

1.4.3 ***Conclusions regarding hypothesis 1***

Hypothesis 1 examined the ability of the BPO prototype to differentiate between clinically meaningful and distinct groups. The clusters which had emerged from the cluster analysis, according to their similarity to the four prototypical domains, were inspected with regard to general functioning, axis I pathology and axis II pathology. Also, the concordance of STIPO based, that is prototype-based, axis II pathology with self-reported axis II pathology was looked at across the three clusters. A clear differentiation between a BPO cluster, high in pathology in general functioning, in axis I and II pathology and a NPO cluster, low in pathology in these areas, could be established. In between these two clusters, an intermediate group was found demonstrating significantly less pathology than the BPO cluster, but also more than the NPO cluster, in particular when focusing on self-harming thoughts and behaviors. In sum, these results confirm the ability of a theory-based prototype of BPO, operationalized by four domains of the STIPO, to differentiate between clinically relevant groups. The first hypothesis was confirmed.

In hypothesis 2 to 5, the psychometric properties of the BPO similarity index will be examined. If the BPO similarity index shows interrater reliability, convergent and incremental validity, this is an important step toward the confirmation of the hypothetical prototype of BPO, and also of the STIPO which is the basis of this BPO prototype.

1.5. Hypothesis 2: Interrater reliability of the BPO prototype

As first inspection of the psychometric qualities of the prototype of BPO, the interrater reliability of the 5-point ratings of the four prototypical domains was computed by examining the intraclass correlation coefficients (ICCs). For this, the independent ratings of two raters were examined for the prototypical domains of 15 randomly chosen cases from the sample. High ICC's (Shrout & Fleiss, 1979) were found, ranging from .95 in the subdomain "Identity - representation of others", .95 in the domain "Object Relations" to .98 in the subdomain "Identity - Coherence and continuity", and 1.0 in "Primitive Defenses". The high interrater reliability lead to the confirmation of the second hypothesis.

1.6. Hypothesis 3: Convergent validity

Following the third hypothesis, we expect the BPO Similarity Index to correlate highly with other measures of axis II pathology (e.g. IIP-PD, SNAP Scales) and with correlates of axis II (e.g. negative temperament and aggression), comparably high as these measures correlate with one another. We also expect the BPO Similarity Index to have an inverse correlation with measures of positive temperament and affect (e.g. SNAP Positive Temperament, BFI agreeableness, PANAS positive affect), comparable in strength to the correlation of these measures with each another. To examine these questions, bivariate correlations were computed between the BPO similarity index and several variables from the self-report instruments, that is IIP-PD, personality disorders scales from the SNAP, temperament scales from the SNAP, PANAS scales, Buss-Durkee Scale and IPO Scales. All variables were tested with regard to normal distribution (Kolmogorov-Smirnov-Test; $p < .05$). As not all variables were normally distributed, Spearman correlations were computed.

Two tables summarize the findings from these analyses: The correlations of the similarity index with axis II symptoms and correlates (e.g. negative temperament) are presented in table 19. In table 20, the correlations between variables of positive temperament and affect with the BPO index are presented.

BPO Index and axis II symptoms

In total, the correlations between the index and the dimensional scores of the SNAP personality disorders scales are significant and moderate to strong, ranging from $r = .32$ to $r = .63$, with the only exception of histrionic personality disorder ($r = .05$). The correlations are comparable to the correlations between the IIP-PD and the personality disorder scales. Note that the highest correlation with any of the different SNAP personality disorder scores can be found with BPD ($r = .63$), almost comparable to the correlation of the IIP-PD with the BPD score ($r = .75$). It is interesting that the index correlates the highest with this particular personality disorder as the BPO index is based on a general personality pathology, not BPD-specific. This might imply that the BPO similarity index taps features that are quite close, or more acute, in the case of BPD. For example, identity diffusion is a central concept to BPO, but in a specific way also to the definition of BPD.

The finding that the BPO index correlates highly with nearly all of the SNAP personality disorder scales shows that the STIPO predicts the whole range of personality disorders although some of the higher-level personality disorders are not thought of as part of BPO. As an example, the BPO prototype does have a significant correlation with the SNAP obsessive-compulsive personality disorder score ($r = .33$), which according to the theory we would not expect (obsessive-compulsive personality disorder being in the neurotic, higher level of personality organization). This implies that the STIPO also proves useful in predicting variance in the higher-level personality disorders.

Dividing the SNAP personality disorder Scales into the A, B and C clusters from the DSM (APA, 1994) does not bring any meaningful differentiation with regard to the correlation with the BPO Index, as the index correlates highly with personality disorders from all of the clusters (e.g. $r = .50$ paranoid personality disorder, $r = .63$ BPD, $r = .56$ dependent personality disorder).

Table 19. Convergent Validity. Correlations between the BPO similarity index, measures of axis II pathology, and correlates of axis II conditions (N=60)

	Correlation with BPO Similarity Index (based on collapsed 1-5 ratings)
AXIS II SYMPTOMS	
SNAP PD Scales (DSM-III-R)	
Paranoid PD	.50***
Schizoid PD	.38**
Schizotypal PD	.51***
Antisocial PD	.45***
Borderline PD	.63***
Narcissistic PD	.35**
Histrionic PD	.05
Avoidant PD	.51***
Dependent PD	.56***
Obsessive-Compulsive PD	.33*
CORRELATES OF AXIS II	
IIP-PD	.46***
PANAS Negative Affect	.61***
PANAS Hostility	.57***
SNAP Negative Temperament	.59***
SNAP Aggression	.35**
SNAP Impulsivity	.40**
SNAP Self-Harm	.74***
Buss-Durkee Irritability	.44***
IPO Aggression	.46***
IPO Primitive Defenses	.56***

*** $p < .001$;** $p < .01$; * $p < .05$

BPO Index and axis II correlates

When examining the relationship of the index with axis II correlates (e.g. the correlations between the BPO index and PANAS "Negative Affect": r= .61), it becomes clear that the index achieves very high correlations with these axis II-relevant scales. In the case of PANAS "Negative Affect" and PANAS

"Hostility", the index' correlation (r = .61; r = .57) is higher than any SNAP personality disorder's correlation with these two scales. This might indicate that a key element being assessed with the BPO prototype is a factor of negative, hostile affect.

Note that the highest correlation of the BPO index with correlates of axis II lies at the SNAP scale "Self-harm" (r =.74). This correlation is higher than the correlations between "Self-harm" and the SNAP personality disorder scales, with the sole exception of BPD (r =.82). Again, this might imply that the BPO Index is somewhat closer associated to BPD and core elements of BPD like self-harming behavior than to the other personality disorders .

As mentioned above, the BPO index correlates higher with PANAS "Negative Affect" (r = .61) than the personality disorder scales do and also than the other measures of axis II do, besides the correlation between the PANAS scales "Negative Affect" and "Hostility" (r = .81) and SNAP "Negative Temperament" (r = .68). Also with regard to the other correlates of axis II, strong and significant correlations can be found with the BPO Index, ranging from r = .35 to r = .74. The relationship between BPO index, PANAS "Negative Affect" and SNAP "Negative Temperament", for instance, is comparable, within a narrow range of r = .59 to r =.68. The correlations between measures of aggression and hostility, that is the SNAP "Aggression" scale, IPO "Aggression", and Buss-Durkee "Irritability" subscale range from r =.64 to r =.73 and are slightly stronger than their association to the BPO Index (r =.35; r = .46; r = .44). This could be explained with the fact that the BPO prototype does not include the STIPO domain "Aggression". The correlations of these variables of axis II symptoms and correlates with each other are summarized in table 23 in the appendix. Overall, the strong and significant correlations of the BPO index with measures assessing negative affect, negative temperament, and hostility as well with the subscale "Self-harm" demonstrate that the index assesses relevant aspects in temperament and affect expected to be core elements of BPO.

BPO similarity index and measures of positive temperament and affect

Table 20 demonstrates that the correlation between the index and the measures of positive temperament as assessed by the SNAP, BFI and PANAS show that the index correlates moderately and significantly with these measures, ranging from r = -.33 to r = -.54. These correlations must be considered "inverse correlations" (as was hypothesized), because they indicate increasing positive temperament with decreasing levels of pathology in the STIPO.

Table 20. Convergent Validity. Correlations between the BPO similarity index and measures of positive temperament (N=60)

	1.	2.	3.	4.	5.	6.	7.	8.
1. BPO Similarity Index	-							
2. SNAP Positive Temperament	-.37**	-						
3. BFI agreeableness	-.35**	.15	-					
4. PANAS positive affect	-.37**	.56***	.28*	-				
5. PANAS joviality	-.45***	.53***	.33**	.88***	-			
6. PANAS self-assurance	-.35**	.60***	.06	.78***	.72**	-		
7. PANAS attentiveness	-.33**	.55***	.30*	.87***	.69**	.61***	-	
8. PANAS serenity	-.54***	.54***	.36**	.72***	.76**	.62***	.65***	-

*** $p < .001$; ** $p < .01$; * $p < .05$

The strongest correlation with the BPO index can be found with PANAS "Serenity" (r = -.54), implying that patients who describe experiencing a lot of serenity are less likely to exhibit pathology in the STIPO via the BPO prototype. The correlation of the BPO index with SNAP "Positive Temperament" (r = -.37) is somewhat lower than the correlation between SNAP "Positive Temperament" and PANAS "Positive Affect", "Self-assurance", Attentiveness", and "Serenity" scales. The association between BPO Index and BFI "Agreeableness" (r = -.36) is stronger than the BFI scale's correlation with the other measures of positive temperament. As there seems to be quite some overlap between the PANAS subscales (r = .61 to r = .88), it is especially interesting to examine the BPO index' correlations with the SNAP (r = -.37) and BFI (r = -.36) as they compare to the PANAS' correlations with these two measures. These correlations range from r = .06 to r = .60, thus showing that the association between the BPO index and these measures is approximately as strong as the correlation of these measures with one another. An example is the PANAS "Joviality" subscale, which has a correlation of $r = -.45$ with the BPO index, of $r = .53$ with the SNAP "Positive Temperament" and of $r = .33$ with the BFI "agreeableness" scale. Especially in the case of the BFI scale, but also regarding the other instruments, the BPO prototype shows sufficient and significant convergent validity.

Overall strong and meaningful correlations are found between the BPO similarity index both with axis II symptoms and correlates as well as with variables expected to correlate inversely with the index. The strength and significance of these correlations and the fact that they compare to the correlations these measures have with one another, lead to the conclusion that the second hypothesis can be confirmed.

1.7. Hypothesis 4: Incremental validity

Following this hypothesis, the incremental validity of the BPO Similarity Index was tested by examining its ability to explain significant portions of variance in axis II symptoms and correlates after the variance explained through an instrument of the Five-Factor-Model of personality (FFM), the BFI-44, has been partialed out. This analysis is of particular interest because part of the methodology of this study is leaning on a study examining a prototype of BPD based on the FFM and the use of it for explaining personality pathology (Trull et al., 2003). Also, the usefulness of the FFM has been questioned for clinical purposes, for example in explaining severe personality disorders. Thus, in this hypothesis, the incremental validity of the theory-based BPO similarity index over the FFM is examined.

Hierarchical regression analyses were computed with the five domains of the BFI-44 entered as a block in the first step of the regression equation and the BPO similarity index as the sole variable in the second step. Various axis II symptoms (e.g. SNAP personality disorder scores) and correlates (e.g. Negative Affect, Self-Harm) served as dependent variables.

Table 21 provides the results from this hierarchical regression analysis. It is apparent from the first column of the table that the *BFI* alone accounts for significant amounts of the variance in the axis II symptom scales (i.e. SNAP personality disorder Scales), ranging from 27 % to 53 % ($p < .001$; $p < .01$).

Also, large parts of the variance (40 % to 65 %; $p < .001$) of axis II correlates like the IIP-PD, the PANAS "Negative Affect" scale, several SNAP scales, the Buss-Durkee "Irritability" scale and IPO scales, was accounted for by the BFI itself. Nevertheless, the *BPO Index* could explain additional significant portions of variance in these variables after the variance explained by the BFI was partialed out. This additional variance explained by the BPO Index ranged from 3 % to 20 % ($p < .001$; $p < .01$; $p < .05$).

Table 21. Incremental validity. Hierarchical regression analyses of BPO similarity index, axis II symptoms, and correlates, controlling for BFI-44 scores (N=60)

	Step 1 BFI-44		Step 2 BPO Similarity Index	
	ΔR^2	ΔF	ΔR^2	ΔF
AXIS II SYMPTOMS				
SNAP PD Scales (DSM-III-R):				
Paranoid PD	**.39*****	.00	.03	.94
Schizoid PD	**.35*****	.00	**.05***	.04
Schizotypal PD	**.41*****	.00	**.05***	.05
Antisocial PD	**.51*****	.00	**.05***	.02
Borderline PD	**.52*****	.00	**.10*****	.00
Narcissistic PD	**.41*****	.00	.04	.06
Histrionic PD	**.45*****	.00	.00	.88
Avoidant PD	**.52*****	.00	**.06****	.01
Dependent PD	**.53*****	.00	**.04***	.05
Obs.-Comp. PD	**.27****	.01	.02	.23
AXIS II CORRELATES				
IIP-PD	**.58 *****	.00	.01	.34
PANAS Negative Affect	**.60*****	.00	**.03***	.04
PANAS Hostility	**.41*****	.00	**.06***	.02
SNAP Neg. Temperament	**.65*****	.00	**.03***	.04
SNAP Aggression	**.53*****	.00	.01	.29
SNAP Self-Harm	**.42*****	.00	**.20*****	.00
Buss-Durkee Irritability	**.60*****	.00	.00	.49
IPO Aggression	**.40*****	.00	**.07****	.01
IPO Primitive Defenses	**.43*****	.00	**.10****	.00

*** $p < .001$; ** $p < .01$; * $p < .05$

Axis II symptoms

In many of the SNAP personality disorder scales the index could explain between 4 % and 10 % after the variance accounted for by the BFI was partialed out. Note that, similar to the correlations found when examining the convergent validity, the largest R square change was found with BPD (10 %; $p < .001$). The personality disorders in which the most variance was explained were avoidant personality disorder (6%, $p < .01$), schizoid, schizotypal and antisocial personality disorders (5%; $p < .05$ in each case). Interestingly, in this analysis no additional variance in the obsessive-compulsive personality disorder was explained through the BPO Index, perhaps indicating a weaker link to this higher order personality disorder than expected based on the earlier analyses (compare convergent validity section). The index did not explain additional significant amounts of variance in the paranoid, narcissistic and histrionic personality disorders, which we anticipated based on our theoretical framework.

Axis II correlates

In most of the hypothesized axis II correlates, the BPO index explained significant additional variance with the exception of the IIP-PD, the SNAP "Aggression" scale and the Buss-Durkee "Irritability" subscale. The largest R square change was found with the SNAP "Self-harm" scale (20%; $p <.001$), again raising the question of a strong link between our BPO prototype and this core element of BPD. Also, in the IPO "Primitive Defenses" scale, 10 % of the variance was explained by the index ($p <.01$). In the scales of PANAS "Negative Affect" and SNAP "Negative Temperament", the index further explained 3% of the variance in both cases ($p <. 05$), as well as it explained additional variance in the PANAS "Hostility" scale (6%; $p <. 05$) and IPO "Aggression" scale (7%; $p <. 01$).

The hierarchical regression analysis was also conducted in the reverse order, that is the BPO index was entered first and then the BFI-44. In this case, the variance explained by the BPO index changed. On average, when the index was entered first, the variance explained was 26% with a range of 12% through 55% ($p < .001$ in all cases but schizoid, narcissistic, obsessive-compulsive personality disorders and SNAP "Aggression", where it was $p < .01$). This nearly compares to the BFI, the average variance explained by which was 47% with a range of 27% through 65%.

It should be noted that the incremental validity of the BPO index does measure up to the results by Trull et al. (2003). The FFM index Trull et al. examined could explain between 1% and 12% of the variance after the variance accounted for by the traditional measures of BPD was removed. Thus, the strength of the BPO index, explaining between 3 % and 20 % of the variance of axis II symptoms and correlates can be considered comparable in strength to the FFM index.

Overall, the significant amounts of variance the BPO index could explain in diverse personality disorder scales and correlates of personality disorders after having accounted for variance explained by the measure of the FFM leads to the conclusion that the BPO index provides significant incremental validity, thus verifying the fourth hypothesis.

1.8. Hypothesis 5: Incremental validity

According to the last hypothesis, based on the fact that the IPO is the self-report precursor of the STIPO, the incremental validity of the BPO similarity index was tested. This was done to examine the incremental validity of the interview measure STIPO (assessed by the similarity index). If the STIPO interview would demonstrate its ability to explain variance in important axis II variables in addition to the self-report instrument, the value of the interview method would be emphasized. Otherwise, the less labor- and time intensive self-report instrument could be given preference over the longer, costlier and more extensive interview.

To examine this important question, hierarchical regression analyses were computed with the five scales of the IPO entered as a block in the first step of the regression and the BPO similarity index as the sole variable in the second step. Various axis II symptoms (e.g. SNAP personality disorder scores) and correlates (e.g. negative affect, self-harm) served as dependent variables.

Table 22 provides the results of a hierarchical regression analysis computed with the IPO, the precursor of the STIPO, as first factor and the BPO similarity index as second factor as well as the various axis II symptoms and correlates as dependent variables. It is apparent from the first column of the table that the *IPO* itself accounts for significant amounts of the variance in the axis II symptom scales (i.e. SNAP personality disorder scales), ranging from 28 % to 73 % ($p < .001$). Also, large parts of the variance (41 % to 75 %; $p < .001$) of axis II correlates like the PANAS "Negative Affect" Scale, several SNAP scales, and the Buss-Durkee "Irritability" subscale, were accounted for by the IPO alone. However, the *BPO Index* could explain additional significant portions of variance in many of these variables after the variance explained by the IPO was partialed out. This additional variance explained by the BPO Index ranged from 3 % to 16 % ($p < .001$; $p < .01$; $p < .05$).

Table 22. Incremental validity -- Hierarchical regression analyses of BPO similarity index, axis II symptoms, and correlates, controlling for IPO scores

	Step 1 IPO		Step 2 BPO Sim Index	
	ΔR^2	ΔF	ΔR^2	ΔF
AXIS II SYMPTOMS				
SNAP PD Scales (DSM-III-R):				
Paranoid PD	**.67*****	.00	.01	.35
Schizoid PD	.13	.20	**.10****	.01
Schizotypal PD	**.67*****	.00	.01	.15
Antisocial PD	**.48*****	.00	.00	.55
Borderline PD	**.73*****	.00	**.03***	.02
Narcissistic PD	**.54*****	.00	.00	.69
Histrionic PD	.14	.15	.03	.16
Avoidant PD	**.28****	.00	**.11****	.00
Dependent PD	**.45*****	.00	**.07****	.01
Obs.-Comp. PD	**.36*****	.00	.00	.70
AXIS II CORRELATES				
IIP-PD	.75 ***	.00	.00	.56
PANAS Negative Affect	**.41*****	.00	**.08****	.01
PANAS Hostility	**.48*****	.00	**.05***	.03
SNAP Negative Temperament	**.64*****	.00	**.05****	.01
SNAP Aggression	.67***	.00	.01	.15
SNAP Self-Harm	**.54*****	.00	**.16*****	.00
Buss-Durkee Irritability	**.59*****	.00	.00	.99

*** $p < .001$; ** $p < .01$; * $p < .05$

Axis II symptoms

In the case of several of the SNAP personality disorder scales, the index could explain between 3 % and 11 % after the variance accounted for by the IPO was partialed out. The largest R square change was found with avoidant personality disorder (11 %; $p < .01$). In BPD, 3 % of the variance could be accounted for by the index after a very large amount of variance (73 %) was already explained by the IPO. In schizoid personality disorder, 10%, and in dependent personality disorder 7 % of the variance were explained by the BPO index. In the remaining SNAP personality disorder scales (paranoid, schizotypal, antisocial, narcissistic, histrionic, obsessive-compulsive personality disorders), no additional variance was explained by the index.

Overall, it becomes clear that the IPO accounts for large amounts of the variance, but the index was able to explain significant additional portions of variance in several personality disorders.

Axis II correlates

In many of the hypothesized axis II correlates, the BPO index explained significant additional variance (between 5% and 16%) after the variance accounted for by the IPO was partialed out. The largest R square change was found with the SNAP "Self-harm" scale (16%; $p < .001$), again raising the question of a strong link between our BPO prototype and this core element of BPD. Also, in the scales PANAS "Negative Affect" and SNAP "Negative Temperament", 8 % and 5 % of the variance was explained by the index. Regarding scales of hostility and irritability, only in the case of PANAS "Hostility" the index explained additional 5 % of the variance, in the cases of SNAP "Aggression" and Buss-Durkee "Irritability", no additional variance was accounted for by the index.

The hierarchical regression analysis was also conducted in the reverse order, that is the BPO index was entered first and then the IPO. In this case, the variance explained by the BPO index changed. On average, when the index was entered first, the variance explained was 25% with a range of 12% through 55% ($p < .001$ in all cases but schizoid, narcissistic, obsessive-compulsive personality disorder, SNAP Aggression, where it was $p < .01$). This does not quite compare to the results of the IPO entered in the first step, the average variance explained by which was 50% with a range of 28% through 75% ($p < .001$ in most cases).

When comparing these results to the results obtained in the third hypothesis, it becomes clear that the incremental validity the BPO index provides is stronger when the first factor is the BFI instead of the IPO. This could be explained through the similar content and theoretical background of STIPO and IPO and confirms the construct validity of these two instruments. Nevertheless, in several personality disorder scales and correlates of personality disorders, the STIPO-derived BPO index could explain significant amounts of variance after having accounted for variance explained by the IPO. This leads to the conclusion that the BPO index provides significant incremental validity over the self-report instrument IPO, thus proving the fourth hypothesis.

1.9. Summary of the results from the quantitative analysis

The goal of this study is to examine the ability of a STIPO-based prototype of Borderline Personality Organization to explain variance in axis II pathology across a sample of patients of different levels of pathology (N=60). For this purpose, an expert-consensus was found as to which of the STIPO domains should be included in a BPO prototype, identifying the domains “Identity - Coherence and continuity”, “Identity - Representation of others”, “Primitive Defenses”, and “Object Relations” as the theoretically most useful indices of BPO when compared to NPO. A hypothesized profile of STIPO scores in these four domains was established, being the BPO prototype. The scores of the 60 patients on the four prototype domains were compared to the prototypical profile by computing the squared Euclidian distance. A resulting BPO similarity index for each of the patients was then compared to several measures of axis I and II pathology as well as correlates of axis II pathology.

The four prototypical domains (i.e. the BPO prototype) were able to discriminate between relevant clinical groups, providing a three-cluster solution. Two of these clusters were statistically significantly different from each other (clusters 1 and 3), while the second cluster was not significantly different from the third, but provided clinically useful information when inspected as separate cluster. The clusters could be described as low-level “BPO cluster”, "intermediate cluster" and "NPO cluster". They were dissimilar on levels of pathology in general functioning, axis I and II symptoms and correlates. The BPO cluster consistently showed more pathology than the other two clusters, the intermediate cluster being slightly more pathological than the NPO cluster and the neurotic cluster being the healthiest on all measures. Only in measures of self-harming tendencies, the intermediate cluster showed more similarity to the BPO cluster than expected, which is a clinically important finding. In sum, the BPO prototype was able to separate the BPO patients in this sample from the NPO patients.

Of the four prototype criteria, the domain "Identity - representation of others" was the most disturbed in all three groups, indicating that this is the most sensitive domain of the BPO prototype. This can be considered to prove that identity diffusion according to Kernberg's theory of personality organization (Kernberg, 1984), in particular difficulties in perceiving and understanding others, is one of the key elements of BPO.

High interrater-reliability for the clinical ratings of the four prototypical domains was found, which is an encouraging finding given the fact that the ratings were based on the clinical 5-point ratings.

The convergent validity of the BPO similarity index could be established. The index correlated significantly with important axis II symptoms (e.g. SNAP borderline and avoidant personality disorder scales) and correlates (e.g. IIP-PD, PANAS "Negative Affect", SNAP "Self-Harm" scale). It also was associated with low levels of positive affect and other measures of positive temperament (e.g. PANAS "Positive Affect" scale). These results correspond to Lenzenweger and colleagues' findings (2001) who found increased negative affect, aggressive dyscontrol and dysphoria as well as low levels of positive affect associated with the IPO scales Identity diffusion, Primitive defenses and Reality Testing. The IPO and STIPO are closely related, the IPO being the self-report precursor of the STIPO. The STIPO-based prototype included "Identity" subscales, "Primitive Defenses" and "Object Relations" although not "Reality Testing". Both the results of Lenzenweger at al.'s study and of this study can be considered as very encouraging findings for the construct validity regarding the concepts of

Kernberg's theory of personality organization, as similar results were found across multiple assessment methods.

Also, the BPO similarity index showed substantial incremental validity when entered into a hierarchical regression with the scales of a measure of the Five-Factor-Model of Personality (BFI-44) entered as first block and the BPO index as second variable. The BPO index was able to account for significant portions of the variance in axis II symptoms (e.g. SNAP BPD scale, SNAP avoidant personality disorder scale) and correlates (e.g. SNAP "Self-Harm" scale, SNAP "Negative Temperament" scale, PANAS "Hostility" scale).

Lastly, the incremental validity of the BPO similarity index was tested by examining its ability to explain additional portions of variance after the scales of the self-report measure IPO had been entered as first block into the hierarchical regression procedure. Again, the index was able to explain additional variance after the IPO in axis II symptoms and correlates. This suggests that the IPO and BPO similarity index (based on the domains of the STIPO) are closely related and assess similar content, confirming the construct validity of the assessed domains. The additionally explained variance importantly verifies the hypothesis that the interview measure STIPO could provide further information over the self-report measure.

2 Qualitative Analysis: Examination of single cases

After the results from the quantitative analysis were presented in the previous section, now four individual cases will be examined. These patients were chosen for a more detailed study as they represent patient groups differing in the levels of pathology and in the fulfillment of the STIPO based prototypical criteria.

The first is a patient at the lower level of Borderline Personality Organization (according to the STIPO level of personality organization "Borderline 2") and fulfills all of the four prototypical criteria. She could be regarded as a typical Borderline Patient and thus, this section should begin with her description. The second is a very low functioning and very disturbed patient, whose personality structure is at the low level of BPO ("Borderline 3") and who clearly fulfills all four of the prototype's criteria. The third patient can be located at a higher level of BPO ("Borderline 1"), fulfilling two of the four prototypical criteria. Finally, the last patient is a patient with Neurotic Personality Organization ("Neurotic 1") who clearly does not fulfill any of the criteria from the prototype of BPO.

The focus of this section is not to provide each patient's detailed history but to show how through the STIPO a "snapshot" of the patient's personality structure can be obtained and how the level of personality organization can be assessed. In comparing the four individual patients, it should become clear how the prototype of BPO discriminates between different patient groups (Normal, Neurotic 1, Neurotic 2, Borderline 1, Borderline 2, Borderline 3) and can contribute to further decisions with regard to the patient's treatment. Also, for each patient, the information obtained from the STIPO will be complemented by comparing it to the results from the self-reports the patient had completed. This will provide an overview of the core elements of each patient's pathology and will show the areas where the different instruments overlap and where their foci of assessment diverge.

2.1. Example of a patient at a low level of BPO

2.1.1 Introduction and history

As the goal of this study is the establishment of a prototype of BPO, a very typical Borderline Personality Disorder patient was chosen for the description of an individual case. This is a 29 year-old female married patient who was hospitalized after an episode of cutting and a situation with severe suicidal ideation and gesture, in which she had held one of her husbands knives against her throat. She had been cutting her arms and legs for approximately 10 years, had several suicide attempts and was diagnosed with BPD four years ago. She had no prior psychiatric diagnoses. She had been in treatment with a cognitive-behavior therapy approach on an outpatient basis for one year, consisting of individual and group sessions that she did not attend regularly. After her past suicide attempts, she had been hospitalized several times for a few days in hospitals for stabilization.

This patient was born and grew up in a US-American town and throughout the last years had a rather diverse series of jobs and engagement in college education. She had taken some trading courses, had established an event marketing company where she had worked as a boss for two years, and most recently had started dentistry training and was a full time student for the last one and a half years. She got married six years ago, had worked in several jobs during the past few years, and her present life situation was slightly unstable as she and her husband had moved from their apartment into part of some relative's house for financial reasons. Her husband, who was reluctant to take on a job, had urged her to this move. This living arrangement was rather unsatisfactory for the patient as it increased her dependence from these relatives and her privacy decreased and thus she reported it as one of many reasons for her suicidal behavior. One might also consider her relationship with her husband, in particular his dominant behavior as another reason for her suicidal ideation and gestures, although she did not explicitly report to suffer from his behavior.

She was an inpatient at the personality disorders specialized unit of New York Presbyterian Hospital for two weeks at the middle of which she agreed to participate in the study and to be interviewed, although she seemed rather suspicious of the study at first. This suspicion waned and during the interview, she presented herself compliant and slightly submissive with little emotional involvement. Mainly when talking about her husband and the present living situation with her parents, her affect got more vivid and she showed a rather disgusted facial expression. Interestingly, after showing such negative affect with respect to her home situation, she repeatedly emphasized her interest to return there as soon as possible. She seemed eager to distance herself from the other patients on the unit and seemed to appreciate having been chosen to participate in the study. Overall, she made the impression of a relatively intelligent, slightly helpless woman and evoked the feeling of sympathy in me, although the naiveté of how she dealt with her seemingly aggressive husband also raised the question of masochistic elements in her personality.

2.1.2 <u>Results of STIPO</u>

The results in the STIPO will be explained in detail for each domain and subdomain separately. In the appendix the STIPO score form shows the individual items. Examples of the individual scores per item (on the 0-2 scale) within each domain will be mentioned in the text and explained. Also, the clinical judgment (on the 1-5 scale) will be provided. The results of this patient can be seen in both rating systems in figure 19, forming her profile. As mentioned above, the clinical judgment, rated on the 1-5 point scale, shown in the graph in the solid line, was used to compare the patient's results to the prototype and to establish her STIPO structural level. The "Impression based on scores", that is the mean scores per domain, consisting of the means of the individual 0-2 point scores per domain, was transformed mathematically to a 1-5 scale in order to enable comparability and is shown in the dotted line in the graph. The mean scores were not used to compare the individual patient's results to the prototype. The discrepancies in the results of the 5-point ratings as opposed to the 3-point ratings (which had been transformed to a 5-point scale) are discussed in chapter 2.1.2.8.

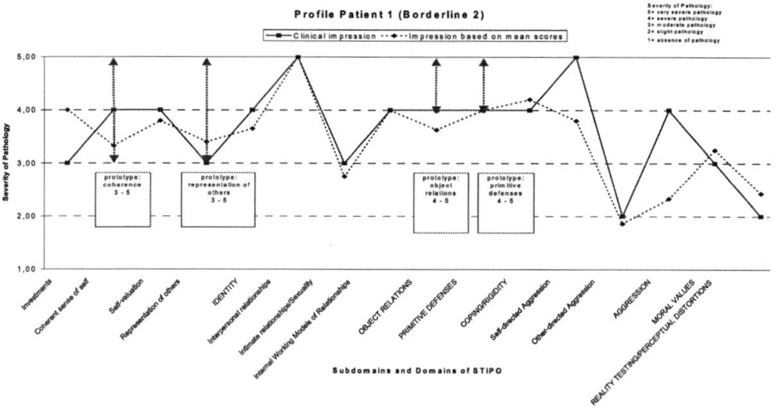

Figure 19. STIPO profile of patient 1 with domains of BPO prototype

2.1.2.1 *Identity*

In the first subdomain "Investments" of the overall domain "Identity", the patient reported having had several jobs and also educational activities. She had gone to college 10 years ago and finished with a liberal arts degree. Within the last five years, she worked for two years in a event marketing company which she had started herself, had been without job or training for several months, and had gone to dentistry school for one and a half years. In between, she also took some trading courses but did not pursue that interest any longer. With regard to effectiveness in work and school, she reported that she had worked below her educational level while working in the event marketing company and that during dentistry school she was told she could do better if she tried (scored both with a 1 on the 0-2 scale). Although she described having been rather reliable and stable in her event marketing company (score of 0), she stated she missed a lot of classes at school due to her emotional difficulties (stability scored with a 1). Notably, she neither enjoyed work or study very much and could not identify any hobbies or interests in her free time which she consistently and seriously pursued, for which a score of 2 was given. In the domain "Investments" an overall score of "3" on the 1 to 5 scale was given, indicating inconsistent and superficial investment in work, studies and recreational interests. This score was chosen because she did report some successful activities in the area of work, but in a position below her educational level and potential. She also did not convey the impression of being very ambitious or interested in her school training, nor having the capacity to enjoy creative interests in her free time.

Asked for a self description in the section "Coherence and continuity of the self", the patient showed some awareness for the two unintegrated sides of herself by asking "Do you want to know about me being functional or not functional?". After this opening , although prompted, she could provide only a few negative examples besides "I am pessimistic" and used several slightly superficial words to describe her character in positive terms. An example for the descriptors were "I am honest, faithful, emotional movies touch me". Thus it can be stated that she showed difficulty in describing herself as a whole object, but she did show a certain degree of reflection regarding her inner life (score of 1). When discussing if she felt that her tastes and opinions were borrowed from others, she mentioned that since her childhood she tried to imitate others and always took on their tastes; for example she even tried to copy her friend's handwriting (score of 2). Regarding the item "Consistency of the self in the present", she reported she did feel different when being with different people and in different situations and that friends would be surprised if they met her in a different context. A score of "2" on the 0-2 scale was given on this item. Overall, this subdomain was scored with a “4”, as this patient's self experience is clearly unstable across time and situations and as noted in the section "Investments", her life goals are inconsistent and unstable.

In the domain “self valuation”, this patient described herself as a person with very low self-esteem which very much depended on the comparison with others (score of 2) and on external feedback (score of 2). She also described feeling superior to others at times; for example to other students at school, therefore a score of 1 was chosen for this item. As she denied that her self-esteem fluctuated overall, and she mainly felt negative about herself and her self-worth, the fluctuation was scored with a “0”; notably here a “0” is not indicating a balanced answer but a consistently negative picture of herself. Overall, she gave the impression of having a rather negative view of herself, of feeling worthless, and of tending to evaluate herself in relation to others. As she reported alternatively feeling superior to others as well, an overall score of “4” was given.

In the subdomain “representations of others”, she was able to convey a sense of the most important attributes of important others, but still gave a vague and unstable, superficial and polarized picture of them, and therefore this domain was rated with an overall “3”. She described her husband and mother with clearly contradicting adjectives (e.g. “my husband is a loving sensitive person but also can be mean”) and in both cases it was obvious that the description was organized around her need-fulfillment. For example, in both cases she described loving and caring persons and complained about her mother being ill and not available to her very much. But due to her ability to nevertheless provide different nuances to the other’s descriptions, these items were scored with a “1”. She denied other people’s opinions having impact on her impression of others, exemplifying this with her resilience to change her opinion on her husband according to her parent’s opinion on him, thus showing some internally determined opinion (score of “0”).

In total, this patient illustrated a high degree of identity diffusion, rated with an overall "4". The very dissimilar, incoherent interests in the field of work and study confirm the lack of integration of life goals and interests and her sense of self and others is clearly instable and superficial.

2.1.2.2 Object Relations

In the domain of Object Relations, the area of "Interpersonal Relationships" is one of the most disturbed domains with this patient. She reported having had no close friends in the last five years and not keeping in touch with any friends from the past. She described living completely fixated on her husband, isolated from friends. After the item "Social isolation" was scored with a "2", none of the other items applied and were skipped. She described having difficulties in the context of work as well (2 in "conflicts at work/school"). Overall, this domain was scored with the most severe score "5".

In the subdomain "Intimate Relationships and Sexuality", the patient spoke about her marriage in which she had been for the last six years. Notably, in her report she seemed very focused in the past (e.g. "It started out wonderfully, I have very happy memories which I will never forget...") and only briefly described clearly chaotic and unsatisfying circumstances in the present. Taking into account the long duration but conflicts in her marriage, the item "history" was rated with a "1". She reported her husband accusing her of being " a big source of stress in his life" and that according to him she should "be happy to have him". On the other hand she had reported supporting her husband financially and enabling him to live with her in part of her parent's house. It became clear that she described an exploitative relationship and the items "interdependence" and "relationship economics" were rated with a "2". Interestingly, she did not clearly object to her husband's opinion, thus strengthening the impression of a masochistic tendency. Further on, she described not being sexually active at the moment, having sexual encounters with her husband only once every few months and expressed the wish "that our sex life were healthier" (score of 1 in "sexual activity"). She stated not being shy about sexuality and being able to integrate love and sex (scores of 0). Overall, this domain was rated with a "2", taking into account her long-lasting relationship on the one hand, but on the other hand the fact that intimacy was limited by conflicts, that she described a lack of reciprocity and because the patient conveyed the impression of dependency from her husband.

In this patient's "Internal Working Models of Relationships", she described frequent shifts in regard for the others ("Empathy" scored with 2). She reinforced the impression of a masochistic, submissive attitude by stating that she did not expect anything good from others and anticipated others to be rude. She also pronounced how disappointed she was about this (2 in "Entitlement"). She stated feeling "internally angry" about her husband not providing for her. Overall, her lack of social relationships and little capacity to sustain interest in others over time, paired with her willingness to live in a relationship revolving about fulfillment of her needs, this section was rated with a "4".

In total, the absence of close friends, the obvious lack of reciprocity in her marriage and her low empathy were rated with an overall "4" in the domain of Object Relations.

2.1.2.3 Primitive Defenses

In rating the section "Primitive Defenses", several clues were found outside of the interview situation itself. The suspicion this patient showed toward the interview and interviewer emphasized her paranoia. She reported having a lot of mistrust toward others, pointing that out as another reason for not having friends (score of 2 in "Paranoia"). She showed a lot of splitting when she was talking about her treatment team as well, which she first referred to as completely incompetent (devaluation), which interestingly was during the time when she was very reluctant to participate in the interview, and at other times she presented herself extremely grateful for the treatment (idealization) . Also, she reported splitting between the different areas of her life and the roles she played in them – at school being a good, friendly student, but at home being unpredictable, for example in her suicide attempts and mood swings. She stated that she used a lot of black and white thinking, with regard to her husband and to goals in her life (score of 2) , but denied any somatization or time-consuming daydreaming (scores of 0 and 1). Asked about her typical behavior when feeling disrespected, she denied provoking people but to withdraw. Importantly, her husband was the major reference person and thus this item was rated with a "1".

As this patient consistently endorsed primitive defenses and reported severe shifts in her perception of self and others, this can be seen as clear evidence for impairment in her life due to the defensive patterns and an overall rating of "4" was chosen for this domain.

2.1.2.4 Coping and Rigidity

In the domain of Advanced Defenses, Coping and Rigidity, the patient was asked for a stressful event in the last five years and described having serious difficulties with debts after a bad investment with her husband. In order to cope with the situation, she reported having slept primarily and trying to ignore it as much as possible (confirming a score of 2 in primitive denial in section "primitive defenses"). On the other hand, she stated not to be able to let go of these thoughts and fears even in moments she could not do anything about them and to tend to obsess about them (score of 2 in suppression). Also, she reported a lot of self-blame and perfectionism when dealing with stressful situations (scores of 2), but did state to be able to take on challenges, especially at school (score of 0) and to be able to multi-task in some situations (score of 1). In total, she gave only few examples of situations in which she used adaptive coping strategies like anticipation, but showed a strong tendency toward rigid, maladaptive coping. A total score of "4" was given.

2.1.2.5 Aggression

In the subdomain "Self-directed Aggression", the patient's cutting and suicidal gesture served as major evidence for serious self-directed aggression and a total score of "5" was given. She had tried to commit suicide several times through overdose and cutting of her wrists (score of 2 in "suicidality") and reported experiencing relief from tension when cutting her arms and legs (2 in "relief").
With regard to "Other-directed Aggression", she denied losing her temper or attacking others (scores of 0) but reported repeatedly having tried to control her husband through threats of self-injury (score of 2). She denied trying to intimidate others but only trying to get her husband's attention through self-directed aggression, which matches the impression of her submissiveness. Overall, her other-directed aggression was rated with a "2". As a total rating of aggression a "4" was given, taking into account the severe aggression directed against herself, which was the reason for several hospitalizations.

2.1.2.6 Moral Values

In the domain "Moral Values", this patient reported primarily being concerned about being caught when doing something wrong instead of following internalized moral values (score of 2) and often stretching the truth when talking about her emotional difficulties (score of 2 in "questionable opportunities"). Although lying to her husband, on the other hand, she described not cheating at school, accepting a bad grade instead and not going through a moral struggle about being honest in this kind of situation (score of 0 in "moral struggle"). This raises the question of a split between the professional and the private world for this patient, which she had mentioned earlier (e.g. "at school I am a good student, I am a hard worker, but at home I am very unpredictable") and which may extend to the moral values she lived in each of the worlds. With regard to her capability of guilt, she reported feeling guilty in situations in which she knew she had done something wrong, but tending to ruminate about the issue and to feel guilty instead of trying to clear the situation up (score of 1 in "guilt"). Overall, she was given a score of "3" in the domain "Moral Values", reflecting her endorsing some unethical behavior (i.e. especially in her private world) and of having a certain degree of moral standards but having difficulty of applying these to guide her behaviors.

2.1.2.7 Reality Testing and Perceptual Distortions

With regard to "Reality Testing", this patient reported some paranoia (e.g. mistrust in her husband; scored with a 1) and overreaction in stressful situations, which she was able to recognize in retrospect. She described some situations that could be rated as dissociation, for example she stated not remembering her wedding day, and therefore not being able to celebrate it. This could also be interpreted as a consequence of the dynamics she lived in her marriage, but she also gave other examples for temporary memory loss and therefore was given a sore of "1". She denied hallucinatory experiences or referential thinking (scores of "0"). In total, a score of "2" was given, indicating mild perceptual distortions with intact reality testing.

2.1.2.8 Comparison of Clinical impression versus item-based impression

With this patient, the results of the 5-point ratings are very close to the 3-point ratings which had been transformed to a 5-point scale for comparability. The largest discrepancies are found in the area "Aggression". In the subdomain "Self-directed aggression", the clinical rating is more than one point higher than the item-based score (5 vs. 3.8). This can be explained with the strong emphasis that is given to several serious suicide attempts in the overall rating of self-directed aggression, whereas the mean score of the items, is lowered due to the lack of other self-directed aggressive behavior (e.g. no self-directed aggressive sexual behavior). Another discrepancy can be found in the overall domain score "Aggression" where the clinical score is more than one point higher than the item-based score (4 vs. 2.33). In this overall clinical judgment, a lot of weight is given to the severe suicide attempts and self-injuring behavior, whereas the mean score, which also takes into account the items assessing other-directed aggression, is lower.

2.1.2.9 Fulfillment of prototypical criteria

This patient fulfills all of the four prototypical criteria. In the domain "Coherent sense of self" a score of "4" was chosen, showing a high degree of identity diffusion, and clearly fulfilling the necessary pathology for the prototype. This patient's "representation of others" is moderately disturbed with a score of "3", indicating a somewhat reflective, but rather superficial picture of important others. In this area, she also fulfills the prototype. In the overall domain of "Object Relations", attachments are few and flawed, mainly circling around need-fulfillment and reflecting the isolation this patient lives in. This domain was scored with a "4", thus fulfilling the necessary level of pathology for the prototype. This is also the case in the domain of "Primitive Defenses", in which a score of "4" reflects consistent endorsement of primitive defenses and clear evidence of impairment in the patient's life due to these defensive patterns. The prototype in this domain is fulfilled. In total, this patient fulfills all of the four prototypical domains, representing a very typical case of group 1a, a lower level BPO group whose pathology lies in all of the investigated areas, that is in identity, object relations, and primitive defenses.

2.1.3 Results of IPO

In the *Inventory of Personality Organization* (IPO) by Clarkin, Foelsch, and Kernberg (2001), this patient consistently reported slightly less pathology in the IPO than the clinical score in the STIPO's corresponding domains. This is a typical discrepancy found between self-report and interview measures. The two greatest discrepancies can be found in the area of "Primitive Defenses" and "Aggression".

Her level of identity diffusion in the IPO at a mean score of 3.29 is rather close to the STIPO mean score of 4.00, indicating a high overlap in self-description and clinical judgment and confirming the similar content of the two instruments. Also in "Moral Values" (IPO mean score 2.09 versus STIPO score 3.00) and in "Reality Testing" (IPO mean score 1.6 versus STIPO score 2.00) the self-reported level of pathology and the clinical rating are rather close to each other. In "Primitive Defenses", we find a rather large discrepancy between self-description (IPO mean score of 2.5) and clinical judgment (STIPO score 4.0). This discrepancy could be interpreted as a lack of awareness when asked about items assessing splitting, externalization and idealization/devaluation or as denial in the self-reported admittance of these traits which could be assessed clinically in the STIPO.

Also in "Aggression", the self-reported score lies at a mean of 2.06, whereas the clinical rating lies at 4.00. Similar to the item-based versus clinical ratings in the STIPO, a possible explanation could be that the STIPO "Aggression" overall rating assigns a rather high score for the repeated serious self-harming or suicidal behavior but the IPO also takes into account a lot of other-directed aggression which affects the mean score.

In total, the IPO results in the primary scales "Identity" and "Reality Testing", and in the secondary scale "Moral Values" correspond highly to the STIPO clinical ratings, whereas the primary scale "Primitive Defenses" and secondary Scale "Aggression" show some divergence, perhaps due to response patterns in self-reports as opposed to a interviewer's clinical rating.

2.1.4 Results of SNAP

A large and diverse amount of information regarding this patient's temperament characteristics and personality pathology can be obtained from the *Schedule for Nonadaptive and Adaptive Personality (SNAP)* by Clark (1993), so it will be looked at in more depth. First, we can examine the patient's Temperament Scales in comparison to the unisex norms of a norm sample of 561 normal adults (Clark et al., 2005). Then, we can compare her Temperament scales to a unisex sample of 143 inpatients (Clark et al., 2005) With regard to the diagnostic scales, we will compare her dimensional personality disorder ratings to the norms of a sample of 345 female college students and to the unisex norms of a sample of 45 inpatients (Clark, 1993).

2.1.4.1 Validity, Trait and Temperament Scales

As we consider this patient a typical Borderline patient, we want to compare her results to healthy individuals and to inpatients. Where do her results fall in relation to normal individuals and also, how do they compare to inpatients?

In figure 20, we can see that in a lot of the validity, trait and temperament scales, her T-Scores, which were calculated based on a college sample, lie outside of the norm range of healthy individuals, but also a few exceptions can be found. "Normal" T-scores range from 35 to 70 in the validity scales, and from 35 to 65 in the temperament and trait scales. They are indicated by the two lines in the figure. T-scores outside of this range are considered unusual.

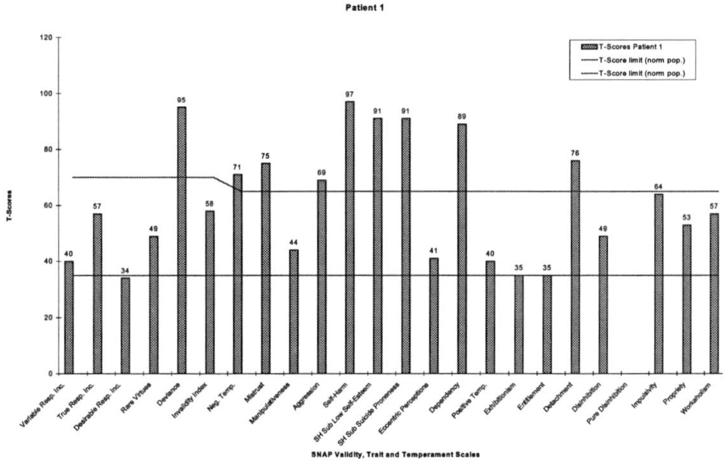

Figure 20. SNAP Temperament scales, comparison to norm T-Scores

Compared to a normal population, in part the results in the validity scales fall into the normal range, but the "Invalidity Index" is in the higher end and the scale "Deviance" outside of the norm range. Thus, the results do not strongly indicate variable response patterns or desirable responses, but have to be interpreted carefully because of the slightly elevated Invalidity Index. Interestingly, this patient does reach a very high score in "Deviance" (T-score of

95), according to which she endorses socially deviant thoughts, feelings and behaviors (for example "I have tried to commit suicide"), which seems very plausible for a patient with a personality disorder and with her history. This elevated score compared to a normal population also stands out when compared to inpatients (figure 21) , where the result in this scale is outside of the norm range of the inpatient sample. The other validity scale means fall into the norm range of the inpatient sample.

Thus, this patient's response patterns do not suggest invalidity, with the exception of deviant thoughts and behaviors, which compared to normal individuals and to inpatients are very strong.

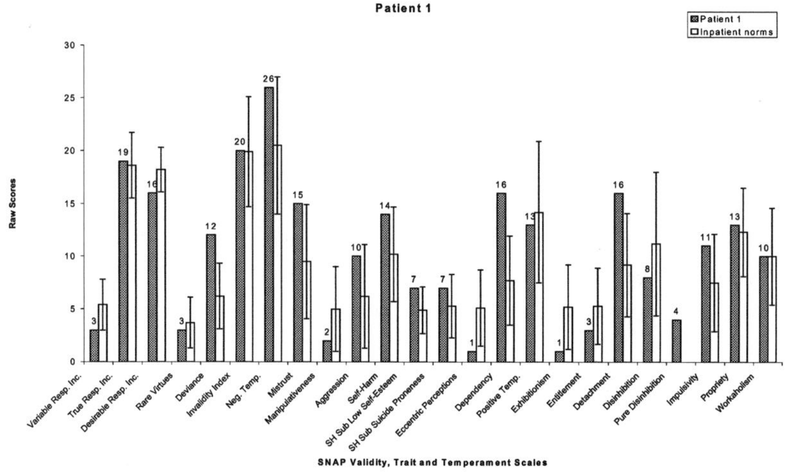

Figure 21. SNAP Temperament scales, comparison to inpatient norms

Within the temperament scales, in comparison to the normal population, the scales "Negative Temperament", "Mistrust", "Aggression", "Self Harm" with subscales "Low Self Esteem" and "Suicide Proneness", "Dependency" and the scale "Detachment" are considered outside of the norm (figure 20). Thus, compared to normal populations, the patient described herself experiencing more negative emotions and to tending to overreact to stresses of daily life and reported high levels of suspicion and hypersensitivity - which matches the paranoid impression in the STIPO. She reports a higher level of anger and aggression and endorses more self-destructive thoughts and behaviors. Her elevated score in the scale "Dependency" confirms the dependency from her husband and parents as it showed in the STIPO, and the social isolation she talked about in the interview is confirmed in an high score in detachment.

As can be seen in figure 21, this patient's raw scores lie within the norms of a clinical population described by Clark (1993), apart from two exceptions. As in the comparison to healthy individuals, her scores in "Dependency" and in "Detachment" fall out of the inpatient norms. This confirms the dependency on a few important people, while being completely isolated from others, that is a severe impairment in object relations as was assessed in the STIPO. The other scores fall into the inpatient norms, albeit the results which stood out compared to normals are still high in relation to inpatients, namely "Negative Temperament", "Mistrust", "Aggression", "Self Harm". In the scale "Exhibitionism" a very low score can be seen. In total, these results, especially the high T-Scores in comparison to the normal population, as well as the fact that most of her results can be found within the norms of a clinical sample, clearly indicate strong pathology in the interpersonal field. Her high scores in negative temperament and mistrust, as well as aggression and self-harm, according to Clark (1993), are strongly related to the DSM diagnoses borderline, paranoid and antisocial personality disorder; whereas high dependency and detachment correspond to dependent, schizoid or avoidant personality disorders.

2.1.4.2 Diagnostic Scales

As mentioned in the previous section, in the diagnostic scales (figure 22), these are the personality disorders where this patient reaches the highest scores in the dimensional ratings of the personality disorders when compared to a female college student sample. The highest dimensional score can be seen in avoidant personality disorder; followed by dependent personality disorder, schizoid personality disorder, borderline personality disorder and paranoid personality disorder. The lowest score can be found in histrionic personality disorder. This profile corresponds to the clinical impression this patient evoked in the STIPO. Her social isolation, coupled with dependence and neediness with regard to her husband, is reflected by a high score in avoidant, schizoid and dependent personality disorders.

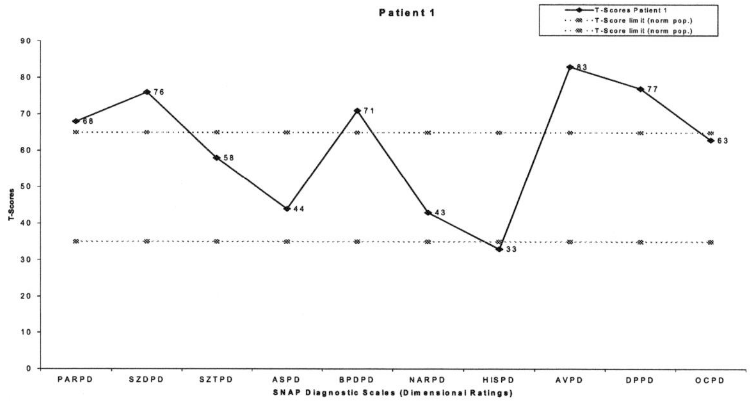

Figure 22. SNAP diagnostic scales (dimensional scores), comparison to norm T-Scores

In comparison to the clinical sample (figure 23), many of her results fall into the inpatient norms but exceed the norm strongly with high scores in avoidant and dependent personality disorders. Also, the scores in borderline and paranoid personality disorders are rather high. Her score in antisocial personality disorder is very low compared to inpatients. The highest scores here are found in avoidant, dependent and borderline personality disorder and thus confirm that this patient clearly has a severe personality disorder, which corresponds to the impression in the STIPO, that is lower level Borderline Personality Organization with strong dependent features.

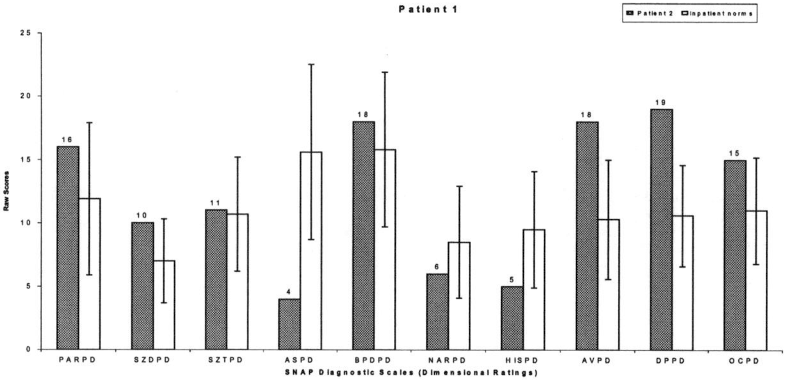

Figure 23. SNAP diagnostic scales (dimensional scores), comparison to inpatient norms

2.1.5 Results of IIP-PD

In the *Inventory of Interpersonal Problems Personality Disorders Scales (IIP-PD)* by Pilkonis et al. (1996) several topics were assessed; interpersonal sensitivity, interpersonal ambivalence, and aggression. This instrument is thought to be a good screening tool for the assessment of personality disorder versus no personality disorder. The patient reached an overall score of 1.89 which is clearly above the cut-off score of 1.1 (Stern et al., 2000) which differentiates between patients who clearly have a personality disorders versus the patients who do not. The high score confirmed that this patient exhibited a high degree of personality pathology, shown by increased interpersonal sensitivity (e.g. "I feel attacked by other people too much"), high interpersonal ambivalence (e.g. "It is hard for me to do what another person wants me to do") and elevated aggression (e.g. "I lose my temper too easily"), and confirms the results from STIPO and SNAP.

2.1.6 Results of BFI-44

In the self-report measure *Big Five Inventory (BFI-44)* by John, Donahue & Kentle (1991), the patient's personality was examined in terms of the Five-Factor-Model of Personality. Compared to norm values from a US-American sample consisting of 711 college students (Benet-Martinez & John, 1998), only the level of "Openness" and level of "Conscientiousness" are in the normal range for this patient. Her results in comparison to the norm sample are shown in figure 24. Finding the level of "Conscientiousness" in the norm range is somewhat unexpected as Borderline patients typically exhibit low levels of "Conscientiousness" and "Agreeableness" (e.g. Clarkin et al., 1993; Costa & McCrae, 1990). Clearly, the level of "Neuroticism" is elevated and outside of the norm. High levels of "Neuroticism" are typical for Personality Disorders, especially BPD (Widiger & Costa, Jr., 1994) and are reflected, for example, in items like "is depressed", "can be tense", "can be moody". The levels of Extraversion and Agreeableness are clearly lower than the norm.

The low level of Extraversion indicates that this patient sees herself as someone who is not very outgoing, enthusiastic or talkative and matches the self-description and social isolation assessed in STIPO and SNAP. Her very low degree of Agreeableness is described in items like "can be rude", "tends to find fault with others" and also is typical for Borderline Personality Disorders and confirms the personality pathology assessed so far.

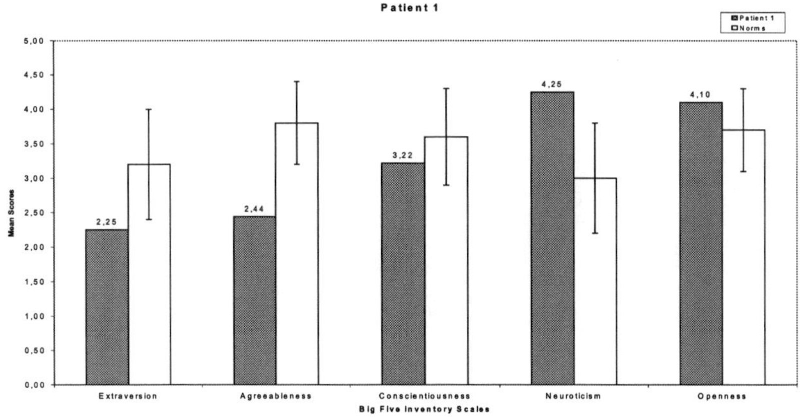

Figure 24. BFI-44 scores, comparison to college norms

2.1.7 Results of PANAS

The Positive and Negative Affect Schedule (PANAS) by Watson, Clark & Tellegen (1988) assessed the overall tendency for Positive and Negative Affect as well as several mood scales like fear, hostility, joviality or serenity. The patient described the degree of experiencing different mood states during the last few weeks by use of a list of adjectives, for example words like "attentive", "fearless" or "angry". Her results can be seen in figure 25, where they are compared to 2076 college students (Watson, Clark, & Harkness, 1994) and indicate a strong tendency toward negative affect and a rather low score in positive affect. In the negative affect subscales "Fear" and "Hostility" she reaches scores that are clearly higher than the norms. In the positive affect subscales, namely in "Joviality" and "Self-assurance" her scores are clearly very much below the norm range.

These results are in line with the results in the other instruments, especially with the "Negative Temperament" or "Aggression" scales in the SNAP, the factor "Neuroticism" in the BFI and with the clinical impression of a patient with high degree of negative affect and aggression in the STIPO.

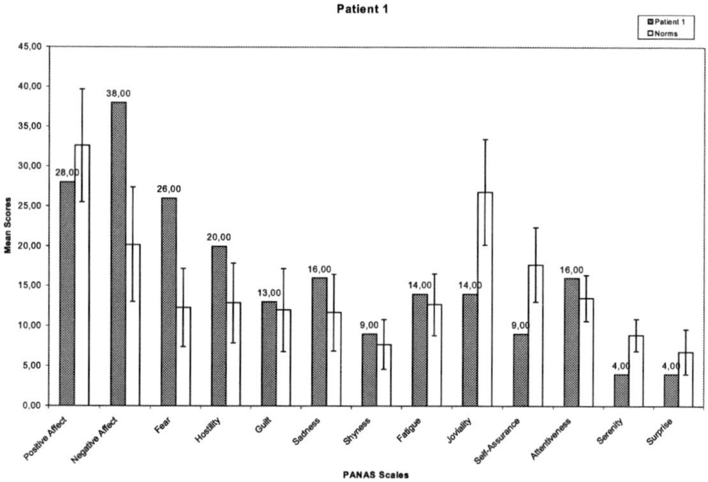

Figure 25. PANAS scales, comparison to student norms

2.1.8 <u>Results of Buss-Durkee-Inventory</u>

In the *Buss-Durkee-Inventory* by Buss und Durkee (1957), this patient reached a rather high degree of irritability when compared to a sample of 74 female students (Buss & Durkee, 1957). The results are presented in figure 26. Her total irritability score is clearly higher than the norm range, also her scores in "Suspicion", "Guilt", "Resentment", "Indirect Hostility", "Negativism" and "Irritability". Interestingly, her results confirm that this patient tends to employ indirect hostility and a negativistic attitude instead of verbal hostility or assault. In these two direct forms of hostility her score lies in the norm range of the student sample. This matches the clinical impression in the STIPO of this patient using more self-directed aggression and not open aggression toward others but instead indirect forms like intimidating behavior, for example threatening her husband through self-injuries. The high score in guilt corresponds to her STIPO-assessed self-recriminative way of experiencing guilt. In total, this patient describes herself as a person with very high levels of irritability, more indirectly aimed at others and a rather high degree of guilt.

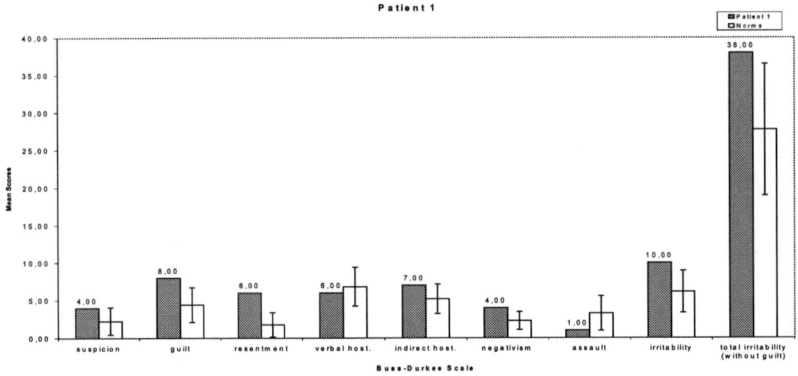

Figure 26. Buss-Durkee Inventory, comparison to student norms

2.1.9 Results of Brief Symptom Inventory

The *Brief Symptom Inventory* by Derogatis (1993) was used as a method to assess other symptoms of psychopathology and to screen for other diagnoses. One of the main questions was how many symptoms from DSM axis I diagnoses the patients from our sample with personality disorders, and who were located in Borderline Personality Organization, would present. Again, we can compare the patient to a healthy sample and to inpatient norms.

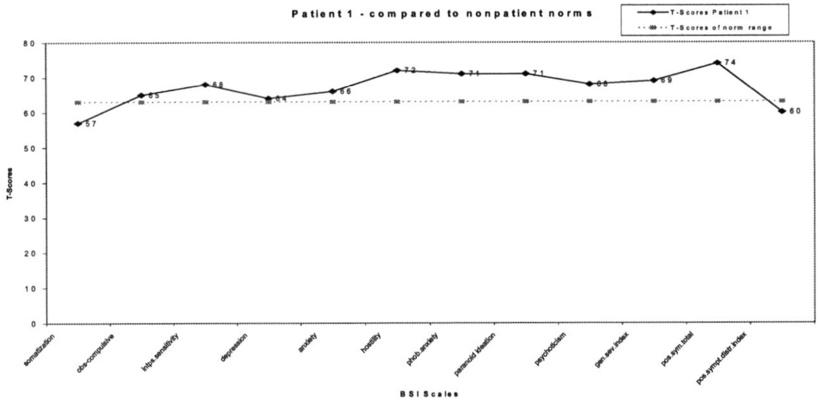

Figure 27. BSI scales, comparison to nonpatient norms

Figure 27 shows her results in comparison to the normal sample, and it becomes clear that her results exceed the clinically relevant levels of T-scores of 63 in all but one case. In the subscale "Somatization", she reaches a score below the cut-off. In the other scales, for example in "Interpersonal Sensitivity", "Hostility", "Phobic Anxiety" and "Paranoid Ideation" her scores are clearly above the borderline of normal T-scores of the healthy sample. The highest score can be found in "Hostility" and "Paranoid Ideation", again confirming the results found so far as having high levels of "Aggression" and "Paranoia". Compared to healthy individuals, she describes enduring a heightened amount of stress ("General Severity Index" T-score: 69) and describes to have a high amount of symptoms ("Positive Symptom Total" T-score: 74), but does not report to suffer from these to a high degree ("Positive Symptom Distress Index" T-score: 60; below the cut-off). In other words, this patient describes various symptoms from axis I diagnoses, for example "Phobic Anxiety", which is in close agreement to the definition of agoraphobia (Derogatis, 1993), as well as symptoms from areas that tap on axis II diagnoses (e.g. "Interpersonal Sensitivity"), but does not report to suffer from these very much.

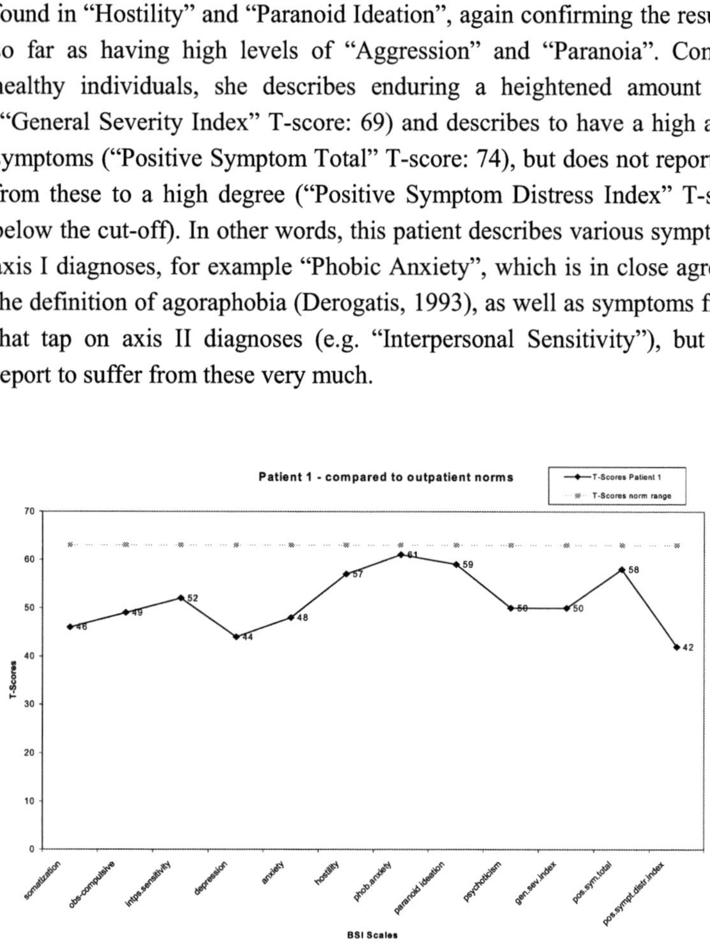

Figure 28. BSI scales, comparison to patient norms

In comparison to a clinical sample (figure 28), her results fit more into the group of psychiatric inpatients. Here her T-scores range between 46 and 59 thus do not exceed the limit of the norm range and do not fulfill the criteria for a "clinical case" as is defined in the manual by Derogatis (1993).The highest score can be found in "Hosility" and "Phobic Anxiety". The "General Severity Index" and "Positive Symptom Distress Index" do not reach a very high level when compared to an inpatient sample.
In total, the fact that this patient's profile matches an inpatient sample better than a sample of healthy individuals confirms that she must be diagnosed and treated like a rather severely disturbed patient. And as this screening instrument shows, she also presents a certain degree of axis I pathology in addition to various interpersonal difficulties which had explained the classification in Borderline Personality Organization. This patient's results show strong comorbidity between axis I and II symptoms.

2.1.10 Summary Patient 1

In sum, this patient appears as a lower level borderline patient (Borderline 2 as assessed with the STIPO) with dependent features. When looking at the clusters as emerged under hypothesis 1, she is part of the cluster 1, subgroup 1a, which is the most disturbed subgroup of BPO patients. This patient's dependent features were seen clinically in the STIPO when the patient described her inability to make decisions and her dependence on her husband ("Object relations") and in the SNAP (temperament scale "Dependency", diagnostic scale "Dependent Personality Disorder"). Other aspects stand out throughout the different diagnostic measures, like social isolation (low score in "Object relations" in STIPO; temperament scale "Detachment" in SNAP, diagnostic scale "Avoidant Personality Disorder" in SNAP), high levels of aggression, primarily self-directed, and hostility ("Self-directed Aggression" in STIPO; "Aggression", "Self-Harm" in SNAP; "hostility" in PANAS, "Irritability" in Buss-Durkee-Inventory) and negative affect ("Negative Temperament" in SNAP; "Negative Affect" in PANAS, "Neuroticism" in BFI). Also the strong self-directed aggression assessed in the STIPO was confirmed in the SNAP (temperament scales "Self-harm", "Suicide Proneness") and to a certain degree in the IPO. Her high degree of identity diffusion was confirmed in the self-report measure IPO, whereas the high level of primitive defenses was lower in the self-report format IPO.

Her problems in representation of others and interpersonal relationships, showing in levels of moderate to severe pathology in the STIPO and IPO, also were assessed in a pathological score in the IIP-PD. An example of coinciding assessments in the STIPO and the self reports is the way the patient described having a very low self-esteem. In the STIPO, she presented severe pathology in her self-valuation which mainly depended on the comparison to others, and in the SNAP subscale " Low self-esteem" she reached a clearly pathological score, as well as a very low score in the PANAS subscale "Self-assurance".

Overall, the key problems with this patient seemed to be her strong identity diffusion, rigid views of herself, dependent features in relation to her husband and social isolation from others. Also, her strong self-directed aggression, shown in several suicide attempts, combined with indirect hostility toward others, as well as interpersonal sensitivity and difficulties in assessing others result in severe complications in the interaction with her environment. The major goals of psychotherapy would be focusing on the identity diffusion, integration of split-off self- and object representations, especially in relation to her husband and also her self-destructive behaviors. A change in the problematical living situation should be also brought about. These goals could be approached with a therapeutic method like Transference-Focused-Psychotherapy.

2.2. Example of a patient at a low level of BPO

2.2.1 Introduction and history

As the first single case was a rather low functioning Borderline patient (BP2), now a very disturbed Borderline patient, located structurally at Borderline 3, will be illustrated. This patient was chosen as she exemplifies the level of a very aggressive and antisocial patient and thus shows the most disturbed end of the Borderline spectrum.

A 33 year-old single female patient, mother of 4 children, was hospitalized after she had gotten involved in a fight with a neighbor with the police having interfered. After it had become clear that she was under the influence of drugs

and that she had had a history of psychiatric hospitalizations she was brought to the New York Presbyterian Hospital for stabilization and detoxification.
This patient was born and grew up in a US city and quit high school at age 15 when she met her first boyfriend and left home. She had a long history of substance abuse (alcohol, marihuana, heroin) which she started consuming at the age of 14. She had been to several psychiatric hospitals after self-destructive behavior and after she was involved in fights and attacks on others, mainly when trying to get money to pay for her drugs and also for her children. Her four children were age 14, 12, 10 and 6 years and had been taken from her after she could not take care of them any longer. The three older children had the same father, who had left the patient after the third child was born, the youngest one's father was a man with whom the patient had had a short-term relationship. At the time of the interview, the patient had a boyfriend, who was active in the crime scene in New York, and with whom she shared an apartment. She has several jobs throughout the years, but no long-term position. Before coming to the hospital, she had not worked as she had become a long-term recipient of social services.

Besides the many hospitalizations, this patient had never gone through individual psychotherapy. During her stay in the hospital, she first went through a detoxification phase from alcohol and marihuana, and was not very interested in participating in group activities or conversations with doctors or social workers. When asked if she would participate in the interview, she clearly was convinced by the money she would be paid after going through the interview and filling out the forms. Nevertheless, she appeared to be interested in the conversation and was able to follow through with the complete interview without any difficulties. For me, it was impressive to see how she did not seem to be touched by any of the events in her life, not even when talking about having her children taken away from her, nor did she seem to feel any guilt when talking about fights or "immoral" behavior like stealing from others. In contrast, she reported freely about these occurrences and seemed rather pleased, for example when meticulously describing how she tried to poison a so-called friend.

2.2.2 ***Results of STIPO***

The results in the STIPO will be explained in detail for each domain and subdomain separately. In the appendix the STIPO score form shows the individual items. Examples of the individual scores per item (on the 0-2 scale) within each domain will be mentioned in the text and explained. Also, the clinical judgment (on the 1-5 scale) will be provided. The results of this patient can be seen in both rating systems in figure 29, forming her profile. As mentioned above, the clinical judgment, rated on the 1-5 point scale, shown in the graph in the solid line, was used to compare the patient's results to the prototype and to establish her STIPO structural level. The "Impression based on scores", that is the mean scores per domain, consisting of the individual items per domain, was transformed mathematically to a 1-5 scale in order to enable comparability and is shown in the dotted line in the graph. The mean scores were not used to compare the individual patient's results to the prototype. The discrepancies in the results of the 5-point ratings as opposed to the 3-point ratings (transformed to a 5-point scale) are discussed in chapter 2.2.2.8.

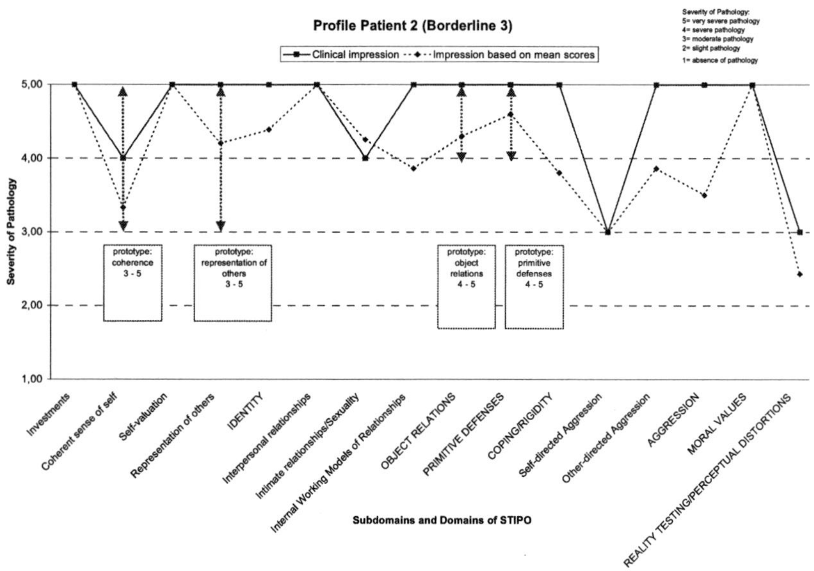

Figure 29. STIPO profile of patient 2 with domains of BPO prototype

2.2.2.1 Identity

In the first subdomain "Investments" of the overall domain "Identity", the patient reported having quit high-school at age 15 without a school-leaving certificate and had taken on only short-term jobs, for example in a supermarket or as a waitress. Throughout the years, she had been financed by her boyfriends and also by her sister, and for the last two years she reported having been on disability due to psychiatric problems. When asked about the jobs she had done for the longest time in the last five years, she said she spent the most time working in a supermarket, assisting in the warehouse. She reported not being effective in the job, having gotten in fights with co-workers and her boss which finally led her to be fired ("effectiveness" score of 2). She missed out a lot of days due to her drug abuse ("stability" score of 2) and said she did not enjoy working at all (score of 2). She could not identify any activities in her free time, her main pastime seemed to be drug use and spending time with others who used as well. Thus, a score of 2 was given for the presence of interests in the free time and the last two items were skipped accordingly. Clearly, an overall score of 5 was given in this section.

Asked for a self description in the section "Coherence and continuity of the self", the patient was able to superficially describe her personality. She used this list of adjectives: "inconsistent, unstable, volatile, difficult, complex, I see the worst in everything, impulsive, witty, smart, dumb, emotional, I am like an actress, sincere". Although using a rather elaborate list of adjectives, when prompted, she could not explain the adjectives further but only could repeat them. As she did not seem to realize that she had described herself in contradictory ways, and also found it difficult to integrate these different aspects of herself or could not elaborate further on them, a score of "2" was given. As she had mentioned in her self-description, concerning consistency across time and situations, it became clear that she experienced herself as a different person a couple of years ago compared to now (2 in "consistency across time) , as well as when she was in a different context, for example at work as opposed to home (2 in "consistent sense of self in present"). She denied taking on tastes and opinions from others (score of 0) and being easily influenced by her partner (score of 0). Overall, she described a poorly integrated and unstable self and was rated with an overall score of 4.

Scoring the domain "self valuation" with this patient was challenging as she reported having nobody but her sister she cared for and thus nobody else existed whom she would compare herself to. Thus, the aspects normally taken into consideration when scoring these items did not easily apply. She did describe comparing herself to her sister a lot and felt she did not measure up to her; thus finding her self-worth very much dependent on her comparison to her sister. Taking into account that nobody else played an important role and she rigidly held on to the view of herself being inferior to her sister, the items "self-valuation" and "negative comparative self valuation" were scored with 2. Nevertheless, she reported that when her sister was absent, her self-esteem fluctuated rapidly (score of 2) and that she felt superior to most people she met (score of 2 in "positive comparative self valuation"). In total, all of the items were scored with a 2 and the overall score of 5 was given due to her highly unrealistic, polarized and rigid views of herself. .

In the subdomain "representations of others", again this patient reported having nobody besides her sister who played an important role for her. She described having difficulties when trying to understand what other people thought or felt, and also what others thought about her (scores of 2 in "assessing others" and "other's judgments"), although she did mention she did not really care about what they thought and did. She denied taking in other people's opinions on potential friends or partners to a high degree, and again, her sister had a certain influence on these choices (score of 1 in "external influence"). Finally, when asked to describe her sister, she portrayed her as a very caring, thoughtful person, who was reliable and intelligent. Confronted about this idealizing description, she was able to present other aspects of her personality, for example overreacting when her children got lively or trying to shut the patient out of her life at times. Nevertheless, she could not integrate these different aspects in order to see her sister as a whole object. She clearly gave a rather need-fulfilling, self-referential description (e.g. "she is a perfect mother, I am not"), but this proved, as had become clear throughout the interview so far, that this was the one person the patient did show some interest in and of whose personality she at least could convey a rough picture. A score of 1 was given for this item and an overall 5 was chosen due to the superficial and chaotic representations of others which clearly were defined by the patient's needs, lack of interest in others and high degree of ignorance.

In total, this patient illustrated a case of severe identity diffusion, rated with an overall 5 in "identity". This patient showed no areas of stability in the sense of self or representation of others and demonstrated no ability to invest. Again, it is astonishing how little concern she showed about herself, her future and her lack of perspective.

2.2.2.2 Object Relations

In the subdomain "Interpersonal Relationships" of "Object Relations", this patient described no relationship which could be considered as a friendship. The only social contacts she had besides her boyfriend and sister were people in the drug scene, and from the people she had kept in touch with throughout the past five years she could not name anyone with whom she had an open caring relationship (score of 2 in "social isolation"). The next three questions were skipped because she had not identified any friendships. As she also reported having repeatedly been involved in animosities and fights at work, the item "conflicts at work" was scored with a 2 and an overall score of 5 was chosen for this subdomain, reflecting the absence of friends and conflicts at work.

In the subdomain "Intimate Relationships and Sexuality", the patient spoke about one longer relationship ten years ago which lasted for five years and about several short relationships since then. The duration of her present relationship was four months and she described a rather aggressive quality with this boyfriend. He had moved in with her three months ago and it seemed like a rather stormy, chaotic relationship. For example, she said "He only moved in with me to live comfortably and to have me do everything for him, but I despise that". She denied loving him or being able to trust him or allow him to trust her (scores of 2 in "history", interdependency"). Also, she described being bored easily by her partners and losing interest in them once she started a relationship with them (score of 2 in "bored"). She reported being sexually active at present and that only sometimes she enjoyed sexuality, but this being the case mainly with men she did not know and not in the context of relationships. This tendency to find satisfaction easier in anonymous encounters than in relationships was scored with a 2. She denied being shy about sex (score of 0 in "sexual inhibition") and said she enjoyed the sensual aspects of sexuality, even more when masturbating than with her partner (score of 1 in "sensuality"), which was also confirmed when she described she found it difficult to combine loving feelings with sex (score of 2 in "love and sex"). Overall, this patient reached a score of 4 in "Intimate and Sexual Relationships". This score takes into account that she had only superficial, non-invested relationships in the past few years, but was able to enjoy sexuality to a certain degree, albeit primarily with anonymous partners.

In this patient's "Internal Working Models of Relationships", she described frequent and drastic shifts in regard for the others (Empathy scored with "2"). Also, she reported showing a high level of entitlement when dealing with other people and feeling disrespected (Entitlement "2"). She denied feeling anxious when excluded from important aspects from other people's lives (score of 0). Overall, her lack of social relationships and little interest in others and her incapability to have empathy with others was rated with an overall score of "5" in this section.

In total, the absence of close friends, the extreme superficiality of object relations, her sole interest in need fulfillment and her lack of empathy lead to an overall score of "5" in the section "Object Relations", reflecting a high degree of pathology.

2.2.2.3 Primitive Defenses

This patient reported very strong use of primitive defenses. For example, she talked about not being able to trust anyone at all out of fear of being exploited (score of 2 in "paranoia"). She openly described how she used externalization (e.g. "of course it is my upbringing and my illness that cause problems in my life!") and behaved erratically ("My boyfriend is always surprised when I do things, he has no idea what to expect from me"). Most of the items were scored with "2". The only exception was the defense mechanism "somatization", in which the patient did not report focusing on rare headaches or other somatic reactions and thus not being impaired to a high degree in her daily life by this tendency (score of 1). Also in the interview situation and interaction with the interviewer, it became clear how this patient used primitive defenses, for example she rapidly switched from finding the interview very appealing ("now that is an interesting question") to very negative ("I have no idea and I am tired about thinking about these stupid questions"; "I don't think that you can understand this"), thus exemplifying the use of "idealization/devaluation".

The pervasive use of primitive defenses obviously interfered with this patient's functioning. She reported the use of defensive operations centering around the mechanism of splitting, for example black and white thinking, in all areas of her life, that is in her relationship, at work, and with friends in the past. Thus, an overall score of "5" was assigned.

2.2.2.4 Coping and Rigidity

In the domain of advanced defenses, "Coping and Rigidity", the patient was asked for a stressful event in the last five years and described difficulties in an abusive relationship two years ago. Her boyfriend at that time was very exploitative and used a lot of violence. She portrayed this time as one of the most strenuous for her to endure. She did report using some proactive planning when seeing difficult times as those coming up (score of 1 in "Anticipation"). She denied being able to suppress thoughts and fears about the situation (score of 2). She illustrated being rather flexible when things she had counted on did not work out (score of 1), and being able to multi-task in many situations, especially in the household (score of 1 in "Multi-Tasking"). Of course, these items have to be regarded carefully, as this patient did not give the impression of making any plans nor of being in any situation where flexibility, spontaneity or shifting sets would be required to a high degree. She strongly agreed to questions assessing her need to be in control and needing things done her way (score of 2 in "control") and also admitted being frightened when challenging situations in private or work life came up (score of 2 in "challenge").
In total, first of all, she gave only weak examples of situations in which she used adaptive coping strategies like anticipation, flexibility or proactive coping. Second, she reported her main coping strategy was using drugs or ignoring difficult situation, thus showing pervasively inflexible and maladaptive coping. A total score of "5" was given.

2.2.2.5 Aggression

In the subdomain "Self-directed Aggression", this patient reported having no suicidal history (score of 0 in "suicidality"). She reported having cut her arms and legs for relief from internal tension several times in the past five years (score of 2 in "relief") and described a high amount of risky situations, primarily in context with her drug use (2 in "risky behavior"). She denied sexual behavior that could be considered aggressive toward herself. A total score of "3" was given.

With regard to "other-directed aggression", she freely reported losing her temper and attacking others often (scores of "2"). The episode that stood out most was when she reported having tried to feed poisoned food both to a female friend who was staying with her as well as to her boyfriend because she suspected them to have an affair with each other. The poisoning was not successful (due to a too low dose), but they were sick for several days and she was neither glad they had survived nor did she feel guilty about it (score of 2 in "attacks on others", "enjoyment of suffering of others"). She was glad she "had taught them a lesson". She denied having sexual behavior that might be dangerous for her partner (score of 0 in "sexual aggression") nor having tried to control anyone through threats of self-injury (score of 0). She also illustrated that she enjoyed intimidating others, for example with verbal aggression or threats (score of 2 in "intimidation") and reported hating several people, for example an old friend who did not return money to her (score of 2 in "hatred").

Overall, her other-directed aggression was rated with a "5". Notably, this patient's aggression is directed primarily toward others, raising the hypothesis of an antisocial personality disorder, as she reported frequent outbursts against others and a pervasive tendency towards severe and dangerous aggression with pleasure in hurting and controlling others. In the total rating of aggression a "5" was given.

2.2.2.6 Moral Values

In the domain "Moral Values", the patient was asked what kept her on the right track when confronted with the opportunity to get away with immoral behavior. The patient clearly denied having any internal sense of right and wrong and stated "I would commit the perfect murder if it existed" (score of 2). Also in the following questions, she reported often exploiting opportunities to her benefit (2 in "questionable opportunities"), exploiting others (score of 2 in "exploitation") and not going through any moral struggle in situations when moral behavior is asked, due to a lack of an internal moral code (2 in "moral struggle"). For example, she said "If I can get away with it, I take money from my parents or sister. But once my sister caught me. She was very mad at me, but I told her I would have returned the money later". Asked if she really would have returned the money, she replied "No, but I always try to make a good impression in front of my sister". Thus, she admitted lying to others in this and other cases, reported having a criminal record due to repeated drug use and involvement in fights and even declared enjoying cruelty, referring to the attempt of poisoning her friend and boyfriend. All items were scored with a "2". With this section it becomes clear that this patient has an antisocial personality proper, as she demonstrates frequent aggressive antisocial behavior, for example stealing from the only person she reported being important to her, that is her sister, and experiencing no guilt or remorse. She also showed poor judgment and failure to learn from experience; for example she did not consider changing her behavior after being caught and punished. As she openly and uninhibitedly talked about antisocial acts and did not question the rightness of these, it is obvious that this patient showed no comprehension of the notion of moral values. The overall section was scored with a "5".

2.2.2.7 Reality Testing and Perceptual Distortions

With regard to "Reality Testing", this patient reported a high degree of paranoia (e.g. not trusting her boyfriend or family; scored with a "2") and severe overreactions in stressful situations. Even in retrospect, she confirmed feeling right about her fears and strong reactions (score of 2 in "overreaction"). The dissociative episodes she referred to could not easily be distinguished from situations being blurred in her memory due to her habitual drug use, and were rated with a "1". Several out-of-body experiences which did not last for a long time were rated with a "1" in "Depersonalization". No bizarre or superstitious thoughts and beliefs, hallucinations or referential thinking were reported. An overall score of "3" was chosen, reflecting moderate perceptual distortions, especially a strong tendency to paranoia and overreaction, and a largely intact ability for reality testing. With this patient, this section provided important information for the differential diagnosis of a psychotic personality disorder, showing that this patient's degree of perceptual distortions explains a clear diagnosis of BPO.

2.2.2.8 Comparison of Clinical impression versus item-based impression

Most of the results of the 5-point ratings are close to the transformed 3-point ratings. All of them range in the moderately to severely disturbed realm (scores of 3 to 5). The largest discrepancies are found in the areas "Internal Working Models of Relationships", "Coping and Rigidity" and "Aggression". The discrepancy in the section "Internal Working Models" (5 versus 3.9) might be explained, as mentioned in the according section, through a low score in "Autonomy of others". The different scores in "Coping" reflect the patient's inability to cope with difficult situations in general (score of 5) and her way of answering to individual items that was scored with a lower, "healthier" score (e.g. score of 0 in "multi-tasking", transformed mean score of 3.8). The results in the individual items must be considered carefully, as, strictly spoken, they do not apply to any of the respondent's life situations. Both in the subdomain "Other-directed aggression" and in the overall score of "Aggression", the clinical rating is more than one point higher than the item-based score (5 vs. 3.8; 5 vs. 3.4). In both cases, the lower item-based mean score is an artifact of several items which were not endorsed by the patient (e.g. "sexual excitement", "dangerous sex"). Overall, without doubt, this is a patient with very strong, nonintegrated aggression, directed especially against others, and therefore requiring such a high score.

2.2.2.9 *Fulfillment of prototypical criteria*

This patient fulfills all of the four prototypical criteria. In the domain "Coherent sense of self" the patient was scored with a "4", showing a high degree of identity diffusion, and clearly fulfilling the necessary pathology for the prototype. This patient's "representation of others" reflects very severe pathology, scored with a "5", indicating that the patient had only very superficial and chaotic pictures of others and also taking into account she had no relationship she showed interest in or tried to understand. In this area, she also fulfills the prototype. In the overall domain of "Object Relations", she reported no attachments of significance or of longer duration and a complete lack of empathy. This domain was scored with a "5", thus fulfilling the necessary level of pathology for the prototype. This is also the case in the domain of "Primitive Defenses", in which a score of "5" reflects a pervasive use of primitive defenses across situations and relationships. The prototype in this domain is completed. In total, this patient fulfills all of the four prototypical domains, representing a severe case of group 1a, whose pathology lies in all of the investigated areas, that is in identity, object relations and primitive defenses. Obviously, this is one of the most disturbed patients, who clearly attains a high level of pathology in all of the relevant areas taken into account in diagnosing BPO (note that all of the STIPO scores lie in the range between moderate and very severe pathology). Moreover, with certainty, a diagnosis of "Antisocial personality disorder proper" can be given, taken into account the severe identity diffusion, persistent splitting mechanisms among others, the lack of empathy, and absence of important others, paired with a total lack of moral values and severe aggression against others.

2.2.3 Results of IPO

In the *Inventory of Personality Organization (IPO)* by Clarkin, Foelsch, and Kernberg (2001), this patient consistently reported slightly less pathology in the IPO than the clinical score in the STIPO's corresponding domains. This is a typical discrepancy found between self-report and interview measures. The greatest discrepancy lies in the domain of "Aggression".

She describes her level of identity diffusion in the IPO at a mean score of 3.55, whereas the clinical judgment in the STIPO was a score of 5.00. Similar results can be found in "Primitive defenses" (IPO mean score 3.69 versus STIPO score 5.00) and in "Moral Values" (IPO mean score 3.45 versus STIPO score 5.00). In these three domains, the self-description of the IPO lies in the range of moderate to severe pathology, whereas in the STIPO the most severe score was given. In "Aggression", the discrepancy was greater (IPO mean score 2.72 versus STIPO mean score 5.00). As mentioned in the respective sections of the STIPO, the patient might not report on several aspects of aggression, perhaps due to items that do not apply to her situation (e.g. situations with coworkers or important others) or due to items assessing self-directed aggression which does not stand in the foreground with this patient. The clinical impression in the STIPO, however, gave the outstandingly aggressive episodes more weight, thus rating aggression with the most severe score, also taking into account the dominating interaction style of the patient. The highest convergence between IPO and STIPO score can be found in the section "Reality Testing", where her IPO score was 2.95 and the STIPO score 3.00.

In total, this patient reports moderate to severe levels of pathology in all of the domains, ranging from mean scores of 2.72 to 3.69. The clinical judgment in all of the domains lies in a more disturbed range, which could be interpreted that more weight was given to outstandingly disturbed episodes and to the clinical impression this patient conveyed in the interview situation.

2.2.4 Results of SNAP

A large and diverse amount of information regarding this patient's temperament characteristics and personality pathology can be obtained from the *Schedule for Nonadaptive and Adaptive Personality (SNAP)* by Clark (1993), so it will be looked at more in depth. First, we can examine the patient's Temperament Scales in comparison to the unisex norms of a norm sample of 561 normal adults (Clark et al., in press). Then, we can compare her Temperament scales to a unisex sample of 143 inpatients (Clark et al., in press). With regard to the diagnostic scales, we will compare her dimensional personality disorder ratings to the norms of a sample of 345 female college students and to the unisex norms of a sample of 45 inpatients (Clark, 1993).

2.2.4.1 Validity, Trait and Temperament Scales

As we have learned from the STIPO, this is a severely disturbed Borderline patient, so we want to regard her results as they compare to the results of healthy individuals and to inpatients. Where do her results fall in relation to normal individuals and also, how do they compare to inpatients?

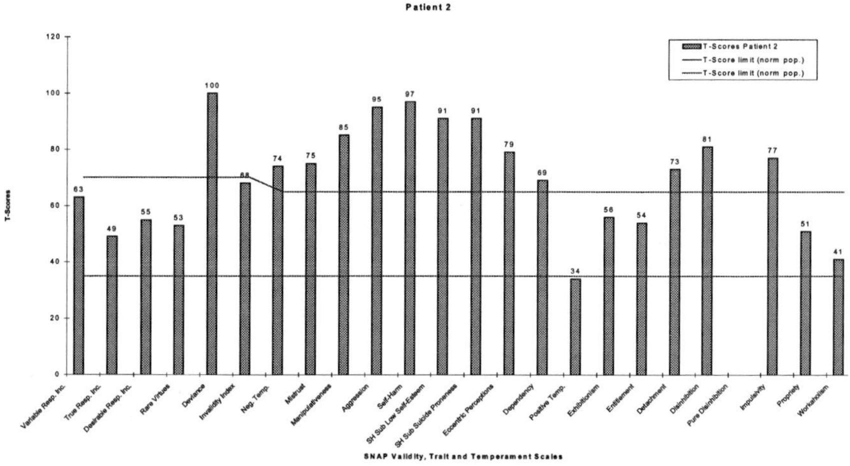

Figure 30. SNAP Temperament scales, comparison to norm T-Scores

In figure 30 we can see that in a lot of the validity, trait and temperament scales, her T-Scores, which were calculated based on a college sample, lie clearly outside of the norm range of healthy individuals, and only a few exceptions can be found. "Normal" T-scores range from 35 to 70 in the validity scales, and from 35 to 65 in the temperament and trait scales. They are indicated by the two lines in the figure. T-scores outside of this range are considered unusual.

Compared to a normal population, in part the results in the validity scales fall into the normal range; but the "invalidity index" is very close to the limit and the scale "Deviance" is far outside of the norm range. Thus, the results do not strongly indicate variable response patterns or desirable responses, but have to interpreted carefully because of the slightly elevated "Invalidity Index". As we have seen with the first patient, this patient reaches a very high score in "Deviance" (T-score of 100), according to which she endorses socially deviant thoughts, feelings and behaviors (for example "I have tried to commit suicide" or "I've gotten into more fights than most people"), which makes a lot of sense with this patient and with her history. This elevated score in "Deviance" compared to a normal population also stands out when compared to inpatients (figure 31) , where the score in this scale is outside of the norm range of the inpatient sample. It is noteworthy that her results in "Variable Response Inconsistency" are also higher than the clinical norm, indicating inconsistent responses, for example answering "yes" to one item and "no" to another item with the same content. The other validity scale means fall into the norm range of the inpatient sample. In total, it should be noted that her score in the overall "Invalidity Index" is elevated and can be seen as a tendency toward invalid responding.

Within the temperament scales, compared to the normal population, all of the scales are outside of the norm. The only exceptions are the scales "Positive Temperament", which can be found at the other end of the norm range, and "Exhibitionism", "Entitlement", "Propriety" and "Workaholism" (figure 30). Thus, compared to normal populations, the patient describes herself as experiencing more negative emotions, tending to overreact to stresses of daily life ("Negative Temperament"), having high levels of suspicion and hypersensitivity ("Mistrust"), and egocentrically exploiting and manipulating others ("Manipulativeness"). Her very high levels of "Aggression" and "Self-

Harm" correspond to the results in the "Aggression" section of the STIPO. She describes herself as having unusual perceptions and beliefs and an atypical view of the world; for example, in items like "I sometimes have the feeling that people or things around me are not real". This matches the moderate degree of pathology in the STIPO domain "Reality Testing and Perceptual Distortions". The social isolation she talked about in the interview is confirmed by a high score in "Detachment". Not surprisingly for a Borderline patient, the level of "Positive Temperament" is lower than the norm and her levels of "Disinhibition" and "Impulsivity" are far outside of the norm range.

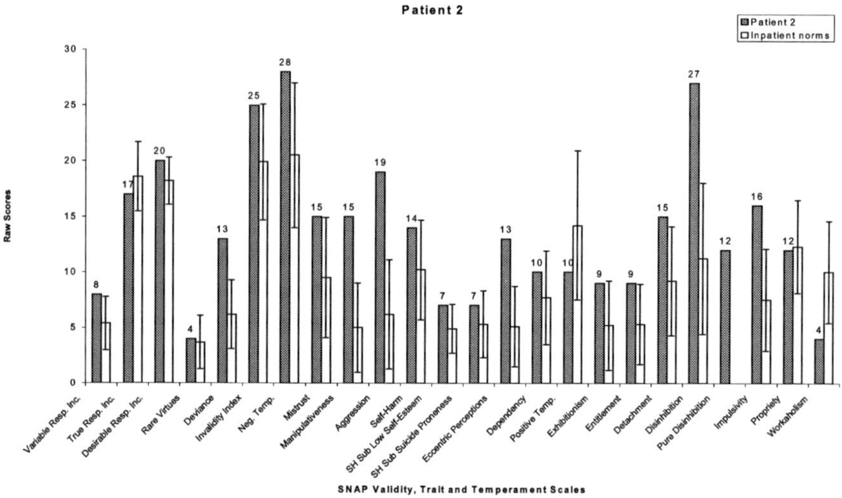

Figure 31. SNAP Temperament scales, comparison to inpatient norms

As can be seen in figure 31, many of this patient's raw scores lie outside of the norm range, even compared to a clinical population described by Clark (1993). Same as in the comparison to healthy individuals, her scores in "Negative Temperament", "Manipulativeness", "Aggression", "Eccentric Perceptions", "Detachment", "Disinhibition" and "Impulsivity" prominently exceed the inpatient norms. Especially the extremely high score in "Disinhibition", reflecting a behavior style of pursuing stimulating experiences without concern for safety or consequences for self and others, matches the antisocial, unempathic impression she gave in the STIPO.

The other scores fall within the inpatient norms; and the results which exceeded those of normals are still very high in relation to inpatients, at the upper end of the standard deviation. In total, these results indicate unusually strong pathology in the interpersonal field, especially the very high T-scores in comparison to a normal population, as well as the fact that many of her results can be found outside of the norms of a clinical sample. As so many of her scales reach a very high score, when regarding the relation to DSM personality disorder diagnoses, now only the three most prominent will be considered. High levels of negative temperament and aggression, as well as disinhibition according to Clark (1993) are strongly related to the DSM diagnoses borderline, antisocial and sadistic personality disorder.

2.2.4.2 Diagnostic Scales

Compared to the temperament scales, the results from the diagnostic scales (figure 32) confirmed the impression that these are the personality disorders where this patient reaches the highest scores. The highest dimensional scores, when compared to a female college student sample, are found in antisocial personality disorder and borderline personality disorder, followed by schizotypal personality disorder, paranoid personality disorder and schizoid personality disorder. All of these scores are outside of the norm range. The score in narcissistic personality disorder is on the transition between norm scores and pathological scores. The lowest scores can be found in histrionic personality disorder and obsessive-compulsive personality disorder. This profile corresponds to the clinical impression this patient evoked in the STIPO. Her strong antisocial and paranoid features, lack of attachments and severe aggression are in compliance with her being located in clusters A and B of the DSM diagnoses.

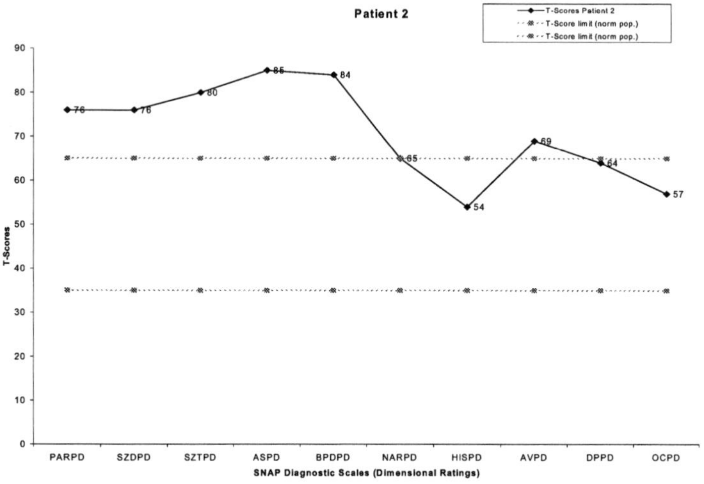

Figure 32. SNAP diagnostic scales (dimensional scores), comparison to norm T-Scores

In comparison to the clinical sample (figure 33), again, her results in the prominent diagnoses are outside the inpatient norms, that is borderline personality disorder, antisocial personality disorder, paranoid personality disorder, schizotypal personality disorder and also narcissistic personality disorder. Even her results in all of the other personality disorders are well above the inpatient mean, but still within the norm range. These very high scores and the amount of comorbid diagnoses confirm that this patient has multiple severe personality disorders. This corresponds to the impression in the STIPO, that of a patient located at a very low level of Borderline Personality Organization, more specifically an antisocial personality disorder.

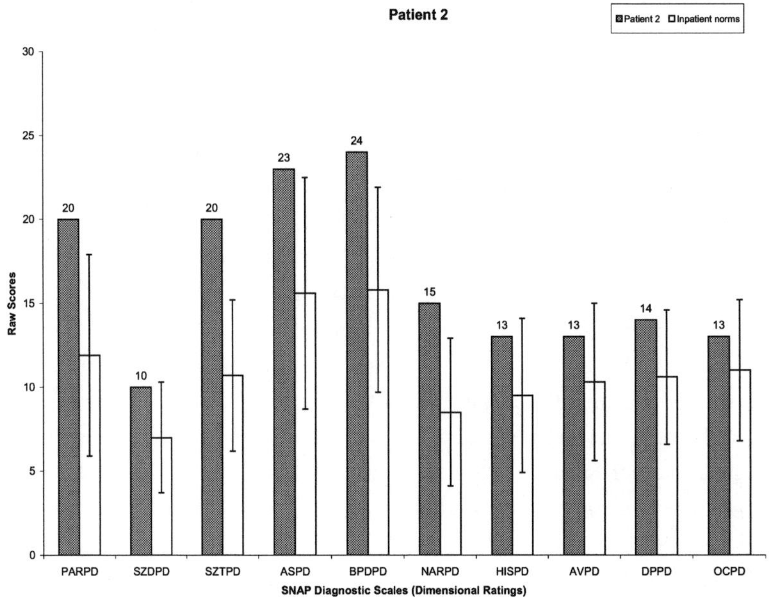

Figure 33. SNAP diagnostic scales (dimensional scores), comparison to inpatient norms

2.2.5 Results of IIP-PD

In the *Inventory of Interpersonal Problems Personality Disorders Scales (IIP-PD)* by Pilkonis (Pilkonis et al., 1996) several topics were assessed, that is interpersonal sensitivity, interpersonal ambivalence, and aggression. This instrument is thought to be a good screening tool for the assessment of personality disorder versus no personality disorder. The patient reached an overall score of 3.71 which is clearly above the cut-off score of 1.1 (Stern et al., 2000) which differentiates between patients who clearly have a personality disorder versus the patients who do not. The high overall score confirms that this patient shows a high degree of personality pathology, shown by increased interpersonal sensitivity (e.g. "I feel attacked by other people too much"), high interpersonal ambivalence (e.g. "It is hard for me to do what another person wants me to do") and elevated aggression (e.g. "I lose my temper too easily"), and confirms the results from STIPO and SNAP.

2.2.6 ***Results of BFI-44***

In the self-report measure *Big Five Inventory (BFI-44)* by John, Donahue & Kentle (1991), the patient's personality was examined in terms of the Five-Factor-Model of Personality. Compared to norm values from a US-American sample consisting of 711 college students (Benet-Martinez & John, 1998), only the level of "Extraversion" and level of "Openness" are in the normal range for this patient. Her results in comparison to the norm sample are shown in figure 34. Thus, she describes herself as someone who is talkative and full of energy ("Extraversion"), also as someone who has a wide range of interests or who is clever, inventive ("Openness"). This does not exactly replicate the impression she gave in the STIPO, but describing herself in such positive terms might point toward her lack of insight and self-awareness. Not surprisingly, her level of "Agreeableness", assessed by items like "likes to be helpful" or "is generally trusting", and her level of "Conscientiousness" are very low and outside of the norm range. This matches the findings that Borderline Patients typically exhibit low levels of "Conscientiousness" and "Agreeableness" (e.g. Costa & McCrae, 1990; Clarkin et al., 1993). Clearly, the level of "Neuroticism" is elevated and outside of the norm. High levels of "Neuroticism" are typical for personality disorders, especially BPD (Widiger & Costa, Jr., 1994) and are reflected, for example, in items like "is depressed", "can be tense", "can be moody".

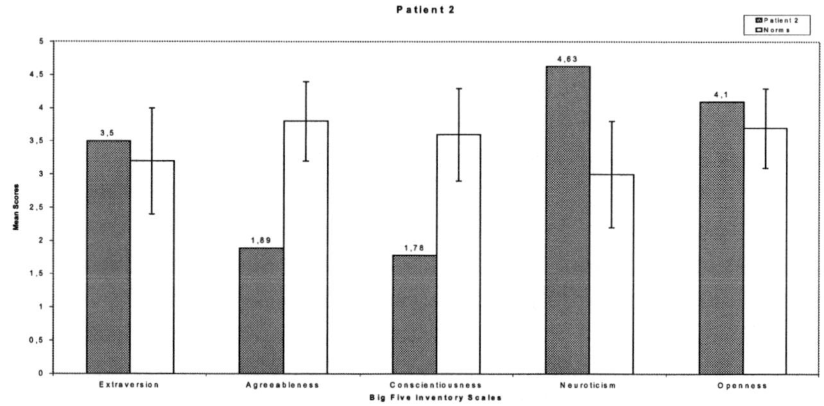

Figure 34. BFI-44 scales, comparison to college norms

2.2.7 Results of PANAS

The *Positive and Negative Affect Schedule (PANAS)* by Watson, Clark & Tellegen (Watson, Clark, & Tellegen, 1988) assessed the overall tendency for positive and negative affect as well as several mood scales like fear, hostility, joviality or serenity. The patient described the degree of experiencing different mood states during the last few weeks by use of a list of adjectives, for example words like "attentive", "fearless" or "angry". Her results can be seen in figure 35, where they are compared to 2076 college students (Watson, Clark, & Harkness, 1994). They indicate a strong tendency toward negative affect and a rather low score in positive affect. In the negative affect subscales "Hostility" and "Guilt" she reaches scores that are clearly higher than the norms. In the positive affect subscales, namely in "Joviality" and "Attentiveness" her scores are clearly very much below the norm range.

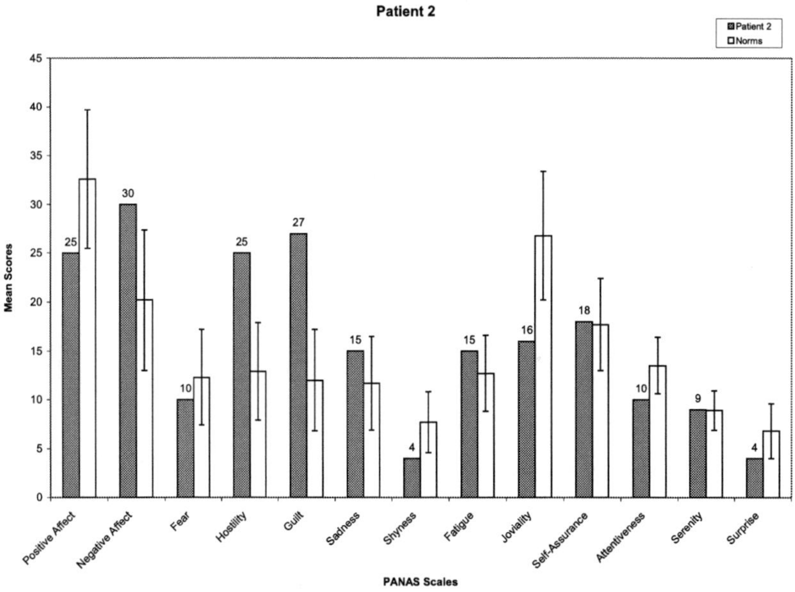

Figure 35. PANAS scales, comparison to student norms

These results are in line with the results in the other instruments, especially with the "Negative Temperament", "Manipulativeness" or "Aggression" scales in the SNAP, the factor "Neuroticism" in the BFI and with the clinical impression of a patient with high degree of negative affect and aggression in the STIPO. Also, the low level of "Attentiveness", assessed through items like "concentrating", "determined", reflects her inability to plan or be concerned about her future, as was shown in the STIPO.

2.2.8 ***Results of Buss-Durkee-Inventory***

In the *Buss-Durkee-Inventory* (1957), this patient showed a high degree of irritability when compared to a sample of 74 female students (Buss & Durkee, 1957). The results are presented in figure 36. Her "Total Irritability" score is clearly higher than the norm range, also her scores in "Suspicion", "Guilt", "Resentment", "Verbal Hostility", "Indirect Hostility", "Negativism", "Assault", and "Irritability". The elevated scores in all of the subscales, including a very high score in "Assault" and "Verbal Hostility" show that this patient is not able to control her anger or hostility at all.

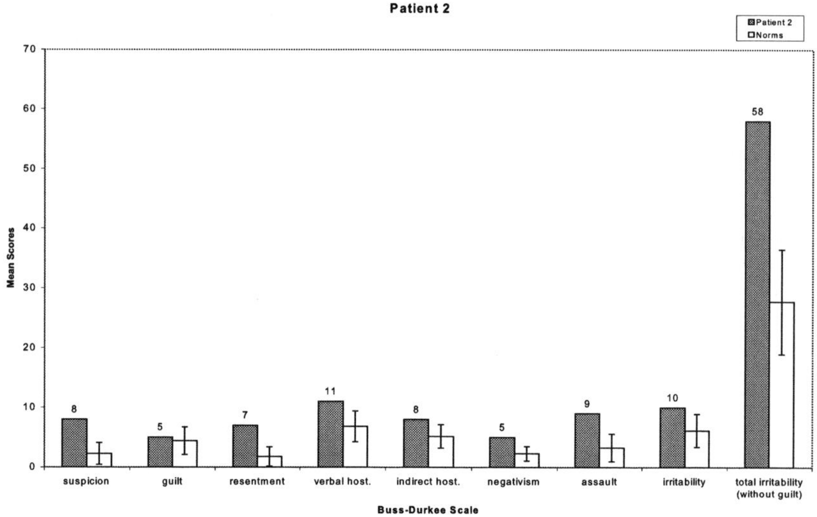

Figure 36. Buss-Durkee Inventory, comparison to student norms

The results from STIPO and SNAP, showing a very antisocial, highly aggressive patient, are confirmed with these results. Also, it is interesting that the only score that lies in the norm range is the score in guilt, indicating that this is not endorsed to a high degree by this patient. As in the STIPO she had described herself as someone who has no capacity for guilt, this low sum score might be another index for the lack of mores and guilt. In total, this patient describes herself as person with very high levels of irritability and hostility, which she openly carries out against others.

2.2.9 Results of Brief Symptom Inventory

The *Brief Symptom Inventory* by Derogatis (1993) was used as a method to assess other symptoms of psychopathology and screen for other diagnoses. One of the questions was how many symptoms from DSM axis I diagnoses the patients from our sample with personality disorders, and who were located in Borderline Personality Organization, would present. Again, we can compare the patient to a healthy sample and to inpatient norms.

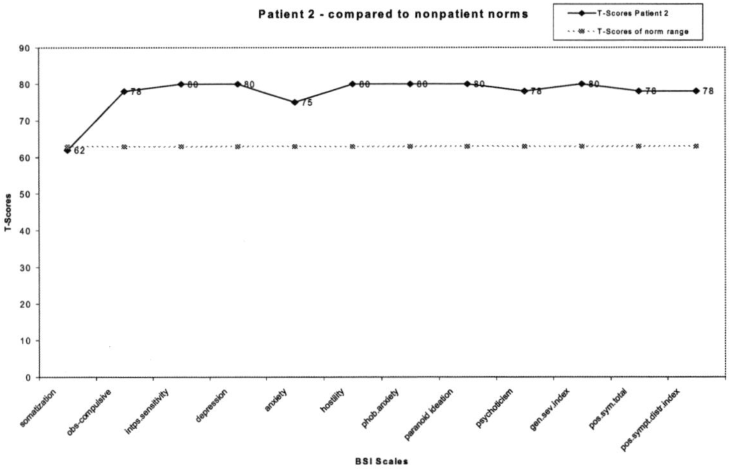

Figure 37. BSI scales, comparison to nonpatient norms

In comparison to the normal sample, her results clearly exceed the clinically relevant levels of T-scores of 63 in all but one case. The T-scores of this patient as they compare to the T-score limit are presented in figure 37. In the subscale "Somatization", she reaches a score very close to the cut-off. In the other scales, for example in "Interpersonal Sensitivity", "Hostility", "Phobic Anxiety", and "Paranoid Ideation", her scores are clearly above the borderline of normal T-scores of the healthy sample. As all of the scales range around a score of 80, it becomes clear that she shows severe pathology in a multitude of symptoms, for example endorsing obsessive-compulsive traits as well as depressive, hostile and paranoid items. Compared to healthy individuals , she described enduring a heightened amount of stress ("General Severity Index" T-score: 80) and having many symptoms ("Positive Symptom Total" T-score: 78), which she suffers from to a high degree ("Positive Symptom Distress Index" T-score: 78). In other words, this patient described various symptoms from axis I diagnoses as well as symptoms from areas that tap on axis II diagnoses (e.g. "Interpersonal Sensitivity"), and one would expect to find several comorbid DSM diagnoses if diagnosed with a more detailed instrument or interview.

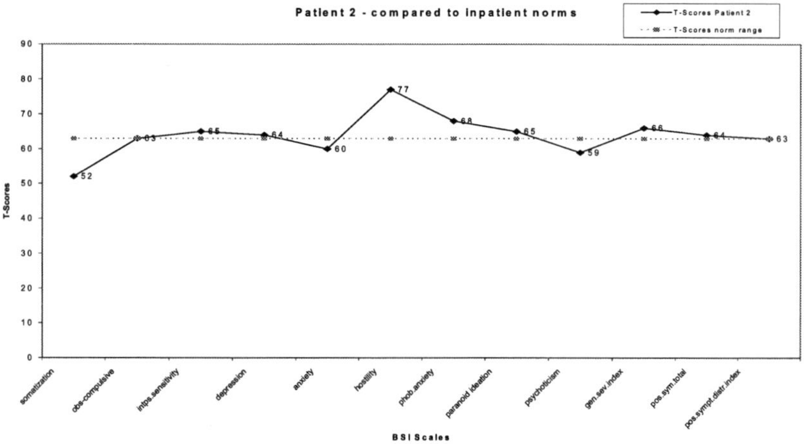

Figure 38. BSI scales, comparison to patient norms

Compared to a sample of inpatients (see figure 38), most of the scales are high, but close to the threshold with two exceptions. Her score in "Hostility" clearly exceeds the norm (T-score of 77) as well as her score in "Phobic Anxiety". Again, she described enduring a heightened amount of stress ("General Severity Index" T-score: 66) and having multiple symptoms ("Positive Symptom Total" T-score: 64), but in this case not to suffer from these to a high degree ("Positive Symptom Distress Index" T-score: 63; exactly at the cut-off). Here, her T-scores range between 52 and 77; and especially in the dimensions "Hostility" and "Phobic anxiety", which is in close agreement to the definition of agoraphobia (Derogatis, 1993), her results fulfill the criteria for a "clinical case" as is defined in the manual by Derogatis (1993). The "General Severity Index" and "Positive Symptom Distress Index" reach slightly elevated levels when compared to an inpatient sample.

In total, the fact that in comparison to a clinical sample her results are at the upper end of the group indicates a rather high number of symptoms and pathology even when compared to psychiatric inpatients. And as this screening instrument shows, she also presents a lot of axis I pathology in addition to the character pathology which had explained the classification in low level Borderline Personality Organization.

2.2.10 ***Summary Patient 2***

Overall, this patient appears as a low level borderline patient (Borderline 3 as assessed with the STIPO). Inspecting the clusters as emerged under hypothesis 1, this patient was located in the same subgroup as the first patient (Cluster 1a, the most disturbed BPO group, very similar to the prototype). As she presented antisocial behavior and complete absence of basic superego functions in the STIPO domains "Moral values " and "Aggression", a diagnosis of an "antisocial personality disorder proper" can be given. This diagnosis was confirmed in the temperament scales of the SNAP (e.g. "Manipulativeness", "Aggression", "Disinhibition") and the SNAP diagnostic scales, in which she reached very high scores in antisocial personality disorder and borderline personality disorder, as well as in several comorbid personality disorders. Her lack of attachments and inability to empathize with others' needs or to show interest in others, reflecting a severe deterioration of internalized object relations, was clinically assessed in the "Object Relations" domain of the STIPO. This was also confirmed in the self-report measures. For example, she reached high scores in the SNAP temperament scales "Detachment" and in "Entitlement". Her severe aggression and hostility, primarily other-directed, was clinically assessed in the STIPO and confirmed in values outside of the norm range in the SNAP scale "Aggression", the PANAS subscale "Hostility", in all of the subscales of the Buss-Durkee-Inventory and the BSI scale "Hostility". Thus, as the aggressive behavior is oriented against others, this patient would fall into the "aggressive" subtype of the antisocial personality disorder as opposed to the more passive parasitic subtype (Henderson, 1939). Furthermore, she presented strong paranoid features, mistrust and pervasive use of primitive defenses in the STIPO (domains "Primitive Defenses" and "Reality Testing"), which could be observed in a heightened score of "Mistrust" and "Eccentric Perceptions" in the SNAP temperament scales, very high scores in the SNAP diagnostic scales schizotypal personality disorder and paranoid personality disorder, as well as high

"Suspicion" in the Buss-Durkee and "Phobic Anxiety" and "Paranoid Ideation" in the BSI. Finally, her high degree of identity diffusion was confirmed to a rather high degree in the self-report measure IPO. Her severe difficulties and lack of interest in understanding others and interacting with them, shown in levels of very severe pathology in the STIPO and IPO, were also assessed in a pathological score in the IIP-PD.

On the whole, this is a very disturbed patient with a severe character pathology. The different instruments clearly came to the same conclusion, showing severe aggressive, narcissistic and paranoid traits, combined with a complete lack of insight, no consciousness of failure and no internalized moral values. As she repeatedly showed ignorance regarding the severity of her situation, presented a strong inability and unwillingness to show interest in others or to empathize with their needs, a very poor perspective for decreasing these difficulties can be given. It can be questioned if this patient would be able to establish a committed relationship to the therapist due to her inability to invest in non-exploitative relationships. Only a very bad prognosis can be given and the likelihood of psychotherapeutic success on an outpatient basis must be questioned. To evaluate the possible success of therapy, according to Kernberg (Kernberg, 1992) several aspects should be considered. The first task of a careful consideration of the diagnosis of antisocial personality disorder compared to prognostically more favorable diagnoses was answered with a clear diagnosis. Secondly, the question about protecting the social environment from the patient is answered positively, that is the children are not under her influence as she no longer has the custody for them. It might be helpful to get in touch with the sister in order to clarify how much she is at risk of being exploited by the patient. Thirdly, as this patient is living on social benefits, a high degree of secondary gain can be postulated which makes realistic conditions for a successful treatment more difficult. In total, extended inpatient treatment specialized on delinquent patients might be taken into consideration for this patient as outpatient treatment will have a very poor perspective.

2.3. Example of a patient at a higher level of BPO

2.3.1 *Introduction and history*

After a relatively disturbed low level borderline patient (BP2) and a very disturbed low functioning BPO patient (BP3) have been presented, now a higher level borderline (BP1) patient will be described to show the complete spectrum of BPO. A 33 year-old single male patient was included in the study and interviewed. He had been sent to the inpatient unit of New York Presbyterian Hosptital by his outpatient therapist after an episode of self-mutilating behavior. He had been given a diagnosis of narcissistic personality disorder, reported a history of bipolar disorder, panic attacks and a recent history of alcohol abuse. The patient had been in one year of outpatient treatment of Transference-Focused Psycho-therapy. Originally born in a South-American country, he had moved to this US-American city at the age of 25 and had been living in the US for 8 years. He lived on his own, and was supported almost totally financially by his parents. His present life situation was not very structured, as he had no permanent job, but was taking on several short-term jobs throughout the last months and was irregularly attending art classes. Recently, he had increasingly been abusing alcohol and explained having several incidents in his life mounting up which led him to the episode of cutting over his entire body in a self-destructive attack.

The patient was very interested in participating in the study and was very engaged during the interview, noticeably trying hard to find the accurate words to describe his difficulties best and having a slightly impressionistic speech style. With regard to my countertransference, he seemed rather likable, but through several comments and some moments of fast changing affect, I got an idea of how periods of stress could let him become very impulsive and difficult to deal with. Also, there was a slightly staged quality to his presentation which emphasized his narcissistic pathology.

2.3.2 *Results of STIPO*

The results in the STIPO will be explained in detail for each domain and subdomain separately. In the appendix the STIPO score form shows the individual items. Examples of the individual scores per item (on the 0-2 scale) within each domain will be mentioned in the text and explained. Also, the clinical judgment (on the 1-5 scale) will be provided. The results of this patient can be seen in both rating systems in figure 39, describing his STIPO profile forming his profile. As mentioned above, the clinical judgment, rated on the 1-5 point scale, shown in the graph in the solid line, was used to compare the patient's results to the prototype and to establish his STIPO structural level. The "Impression based on scores", that is the mean scores per domain, consisting of the individual items per domain, is shown in the dotted line in the graph (transformed to a 1-5 scale) and was not used to compare the individual patient's results to the prototype. The discrepancies in the results of the 5-point ratings as opposed to the 3-point ratings (which had been transformed to a 5-point scale) are discussed in chapter 2.3.2.8.

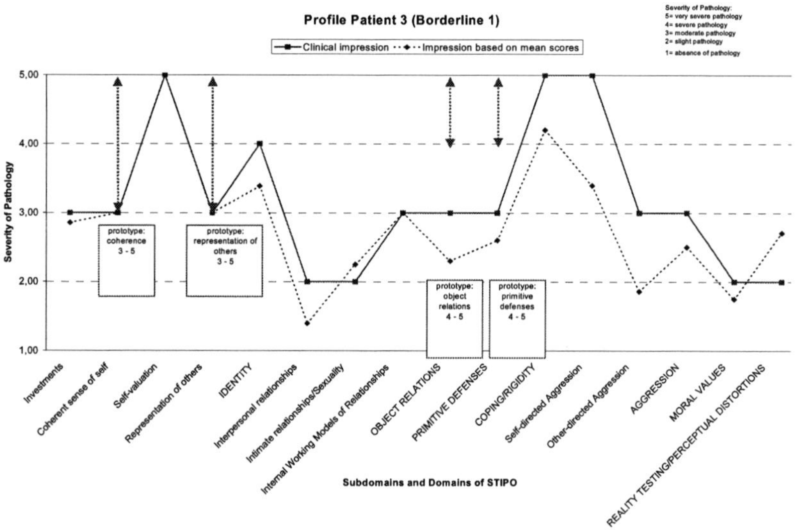

Figure 39. STIPO profile of patient 3 with domains of BPO prototype

2.3.2.1 Identity

In the first subdomain "Investments" of the overall domain "Identity", the patient described not committing continuously to any study or work or recreational interests. For several years, he had been taking art classes, had been a part-time art student and had been working occasionally at a catering company. Overall, he did not support himself entirely through his work as his parents supported him to a high degree financially. Also, he described having been ill for a month with a flu, the seriousness of which might be questioned, and reported not being able to do anything during this time as a consequence. A score of 1 in "effectiveness" and of 2 in "stability" was chosen. Nevertheless, he said he enjoyed his work and art classes and spent some of his free time with several rather fast changing projects like writing poetry and home decoration. The domain "investments" was scored a 3, indicating inconsistent and superficial investment in work, studies and recreational interests.

Regarding one of the core questions in the section "coherence and continuity of the self", the patient gave a slightly incoherent self description, using opposite adjectives to describe himself, for example "I am very trustworthy; I am not one-hundert-percent reliable", and was not concerned about the contradictions. He showed some difficulties in describing himself more elaborately than with a list of adjectives; nevertheless, he showed some sense of reflection on his inner mental life by using descriptions like "I am complicated". Also, some of his statements reflected a narcissistic attitude, for example "I am very interesting to talk to; other people come up to talk to me about their problems or crises". A score of 1 was given in "self-description". Asked about if he was afraid of losing himself in an intimate relationship, he replied having the problem of developing a sort of codependence in his relationships and giving up his own interests in his relationships (score of 2 in "self- in intimate relationship"). Overall, this domain was scored with a "3", rating this patient's sense of self being unstable across time and situations.

In the domain "self valuation", this patient described that his self-valuation changed extremely in response to comparing himself to others and to external feedback (score of 2 in "external influence") , thus presenting his self-esteem as fluctuating. Nevertheless he reported feeling superior to most people he met and having been told by others to be arrogant and to have a too high opinion of himself, achieving a score of 2 in "positive comparative self valuation". Overall, his presentation gave the impression of him having an unintegrated picture of himself and his self-valuation and that he was narcissistically holding on to a rigid and polarized positive view of himself. Thus, this domain was scored with the most severe score, a "5".

His "representations of others" were unstable, superficial and polarized, although he did convey a sense of the major characteristics of others. Thus, a score of "3" was chosen. For example he described his ex-girlfriend in a clearly idealizing manner ("She is a great person; she is witty, smart, talented, funny, active, committed") and gave a rather devaluing picture of his mother (e.g. "She gives up on life consciously; she is very sick; she is fearful of change"), but in her case he was able to name a couple of positive aspects of her personality ("She is giving; she is sensitive and very attached to the family"). The description of the ex-partner was scored with a 2, the description of the mother with a 1. The patient described his former partner in a very idealizing and submissive way, and throughout the interview, a lot of the questions led back to the topic of the girlfriend, at one occasion he mentioned "we belong together". This could be interpreted as a rather clinging attachment, but taking into account his narcissistic pathology, it rather should be regarded as an entitled attitude, in the sense of having the right to be in this relationship and having rather high expectations from his partner.

Summarizing this patient's identity diffusion, instability in self representation, object representation and difficulties of seeing others as whole objects, a score of "4" was chosen to reflect rather severe identity pathology.

2.3.2.2 Object Relations

In the domain of Object Relations, the area of "Interpersonal Relationships" was one of the most stable domains with this patient. The patient reported having a few close friends, with whom he had kept in touch over many years and reciprocally shared personal aspects of their lives ("social isolation": 0). He denied having problems with friends or coworkers ("problems/volatility":0) , although he did state having difficulties staying in touch with the majority of his friends ("stability": 1). Overall, this domain was scored with a "2".

Regarding his "Intimate Relationships and Sexuality", the patient reported having had a long-lasting, overall harmonious relationship for nine years, but talked about it being flawed and lacking reciprocity in terms of openness and interdependence ("intimacy/interdependence": 1). He reported some difficulties with sexual satisfaction within his relationships ("sexual activity": 2), but described himself as being able to combine loving feelings with sexual experiences ("love and sex": 0). Thus, the summed impression was rated with a

"2", taking into account the patient's ability to form a long-term relationship and considering some conflicts within this area.

In this patient's "Internal Working Models of Relationships", it clearly can be seen that he has a very narcissistic attitude, showing disrespect of the autonomy of others, especially with regard to his ex-girlfriend's life ("autonomy of others": 2), and a rather severe degree of entitlement. For example, he described his ex-girlfriend as not taking care of him sufficiently whenever he was ill, using a very entitled tone of voice. Also, he reported his friends having accused him of being selfish (score of 1 in "entitlement"). The impression this patient conveyed was a clearly limited capacity of empathy (score of 1 in "empathy") and a tendency to view relationships in terms of need-fulfillment and therefore was scored with a "3". In summary, his present but flawed attachments and low empathy were rated with an overall "3" in the domain of Object Relations.

2.3.2.3 Primitive Defenses

The patient reported a mixed pattern of endorsement of Primitive Defenses and was rated with a score of "3". For example, he reported keeping personal information away from others out of strong fears of being exploited; thus exhibiting paranoia (score of 2). He also presented himself as using a lot of black and white thinking (score of 2), but denied externalizing his problems ("I try to take on responsibility for my behavior"). He reported somatizing rather strongly, for example he reported suffering from nausea, stomach aches and colds when under stress. A score of 2 was chosen for this item. Asked about erratic behavior, he replied that people knew what to expect from him, and were not surprised by his behavior. The implication might be that his environment had gotten used to behavior like his self-destructive behavior. It was not an easy task to evaluate this patient's use of primitive defenses, as he presented himself rather stable, for example denied idealization or devaluation of people or erratic behavior, but on the other hand reported very strong and severe, mainly self-directed outbursts. In rating the patient's overall use of primitive defenses, the clinical impression was that this patient uses primitive defenses to some degree, but his daily life functioning was not extremely impaired by this use. Therefore, this section was rated with a "3".

2.3.2.4 Coping and Rigidity

The field of advanced defenses, "Coping and Rigidity", is one of the most severely disturbed areas with this patient. He showed nearly no flexibility in dealing with stressors, describing his major coping strategies as using alcohol or cutting and he also endorsed perfectionism (score of 2) and extreme worrying (score of 2). Throughout the interview, it became clear that the cutting episode might have been related to the fact that it was the day after his long-term girlfriend's birthday, and the patient was not invited to the birthday party. One might expect this to be very humiliating for the patient, although he denied the impact of this event verbally. In sum, his maladaptive coping was scored with "5".

2.3.2.5 Aggression

With respect to "Self-directed Aggression", the patient's cutting episode, which was one among others, clearly accounted for a maximum degree of pathology and was scored accordingly with a "5". He also reported exhibiting risky behavior (score of 2), drug use and two suicide attempts ("suicidality": 2). It was difficult to estimate how much the suicide attempts might be judged as a parasuicides as he described having combined two incompatible medications and going to the emergency room on his own. Nevertheless, as he emphasized the events as suicide attempts, they were considered as severe acts of self-directed aggression.

In terms of "Other-directed Aggression", he conveyed the impression of using less overt aggression toward others but more passive-aggressive behavior. For example, he stated he often used the threat of self-injury to control his ex-girlfriend (score of 2). He also reported poorly integrated feelings of hatred toward his father (score of 1). This section was rated with a "3", emphasizing the controlling and passive-aggressive character of his behaviors. Overall, the domain of aggression was rated as a "3", reflecting his primarily self-directed, and rather intense aggression, but taking into consideration that the acts of aggression as a whole did not seem to be life-threatening.

2.3.2.6 Moral Values

This patient's "Moral Values" seemed to be intact to a certain degree, as he reported engaging in some immoral behavior (score of 1 in "questionable opportunities"), but overall having the capacity of guilt and trying to make amends. He reported having twisted the facts in front of his therapist and not telling him the full extent of his alcohol abuse and about other symptoms ("lying/deceit": 1). On the other hand, he stated „If I do something bad, I let it eat away at me for years" and described his tendency of sometimes having self-recriminative thoughts instead of clearing up the affected situation (score of 1 in "guilt"). In total, especially considering the absence of antisocial behavior, this section was scored with a "2".

2.3.2.7 Reality Testing and Perceptual Distortions

With regard to "Reality Testing", this patient described several episodes which could be rated as dissociative episodes (score of 1 in "dissociation"), and situations in which he clearly overreacted, but did convey the impression to be able to see that he overreacted in retrospect ("overreaction": 1). He reported no bizarre thoughts, hallucinatory experiences or referential thinking (scores of 0). The episodes he reported, for example the impulsive cutting attack, which he did not remember, can be interpreted as dissociative episodes. Also, he acknowledged that others might regard his cutting as bizarre but declared he felt ashamed of it. Overall, "Reality Testing and Perceptual Distortions" were rated as "2", indicating mild perceptual distortions with intact reality testing.

2.3.2.8 Comparison of Clinical impression versus item-based impression

With this patient, the results of the 5-point ratings are very close to the 3-point ratings. The largest discrepancies are found in the area "Aggression". Both in "Self-directed aggression" and in "other-directed aggression", the clinical score is more than one point higher than the item-based mean score. As explained in the domain "Aggression", this patient used a lot of passive-aggressive behavior and ego-syntonic aggression, so one might expect him to report less aggression than would be rated clinically.

2.3.2.9 Fulfillment of prototypical criteria

This patient fulfills two of the four prototypical criteria. In the domain "coherent sense of self" the patient was scored with a "3", showing a moderate degree of identity diffusion, and fulfilling the necessary pathology for the prototype. His "representation of others" is moderately disturbed with a score of "3", indicating a somewhat reflective, but rather superficial picture of important others. In this area, he also fulfills the prototype. In the overall domain of "Object Relations", attachments are present, but flawed and organized around his need-fulfillment. This level of pathology is reflected in the score of "3" and does not fulfill the necessary degree of disturbance for the prototype. This is also the case in the domain of "Primitive Defenses", which he uses to some extent, but which are not impairing his life to such a degree as required for the fulfillment of the prototype in this domain. In total, this patient fulfills two of the four prototypical domains, representing a typical case of Group 1c, a slightly higher-level subgroup of the overall group 1 (primarily STIPO level BP1), whose pathology lies for the most part in the area of identity and less in the domains of object relations and primitive defenses.

2.3.3 Results of IPO

In the *Inventory of Personality Organization (IPO)* by Clarkin, Foelsch, and Kernberg (2001), this patient consistently reported slightly less pathology in the IPO than the clinical score in the STIPO's corresponding domains. This is a typical discrepancy found between self-report and interview measures. The two greatest discrepancies can be found in the domains of "Identity" and "Aggression". He described his level of identity diffusion in the IPO at a mean score of 2.57, as opposed to the clinical judgment in the STIPO at 4.00. In "Aggression", the self-reported score lies at a mean of 1.39, whereas the clinical judgment lies at 3.00. As to the domain of "Primitive Defenses", the self-report domain mean score of 2.31 is rather close to the clinical score of 3.00; the "Moral Values" self reported mean score of 2.09 is nearly identical with the clinical score of 2.00; and at last, in "Reality Testing", the self reported mean score of 1.35 is close to the clinical score of 2.00. Possible explanations for the discrepancies might be seen in a lack of insight (e.g. for the difficulties in describing and assessing others), in a tendency to reply in a socially desired way and in the fact that the patient conveyed the impression throughout the interview of using a lot of ego-syntonic aggression.

2.3.4 Results of SNAP

A large and diverse amount of information regarding this patient's temperament characteristics and personality pathology can be obtained from the *Schedule for*

Nonadaptive and Adaptive Personality (SNAP) by Clark (1993), so it will be looked at more in depth. First, we can examine the patient's temperament scales in comparison to the unisex norms of a norm sample of 561 normal adults (Clark et al., in press). Then, we can compare his temperament scales to a unisex sample of 143 inpatients (Clark et al., in press). With regard to the diagnostic scales, we will compare his dimensional personality disorder ratings to the norms of a sample of 216 male college students and to the unisex norms of a sample of 45 inpatients (Clark, 1993).

2.3.4.1 <u>*Validity, Trait and Temperament Scales*</u>

As this patient is in the higher realm of BPO, it is of high interest to regard his results in comparison to healthy individuals and to inpatients. Are his results more typical for normal individuals or for inpatients?

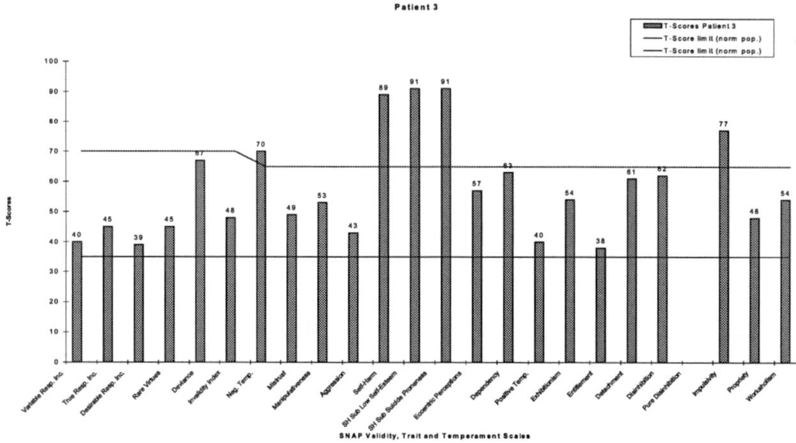

Figure 40. SNAP Temperament scales, comparison to norm T-Scores

First, as shown in figure 40, in many of the validity, trait and temperament scales, his T-Scores, which were calculated based on a college sample, lie within the norm range of healthy individuals, but also show a few strong exceptions. "Normal" T-scores range from 35 to 70 in the validity scales, and from 35 to 65 in the temperament and trait scales. They are indicated by the two lines in the figure. T-scores outside of this range are considered unusual.

Compared to a normal population, the results in the validity scales fall into the normal range and therefore do not indicate notably variable response patterns or desirable responses. Interestingly, this patient does reach a very high score in "Deviance", according to which he endorses socially deviant thoughts, feelings and behaviors (for example "I have tried to commit suicide"), which – as with the first two patients – seems very plausible for a patient with a personality disorder and with his history. This elevated score in a normal population does exceed the norms anymore when comparing his results to inpatients (figure 41) , where this scale and also the other validity scale means can be located within the norm range of the inpatient sample. Thus, his results lie in the higher end of the norm range of healthy individuals, but also fall into the lower range of the typical results for inpatients, which can be interpreted as results of a higher functioning inpatient.

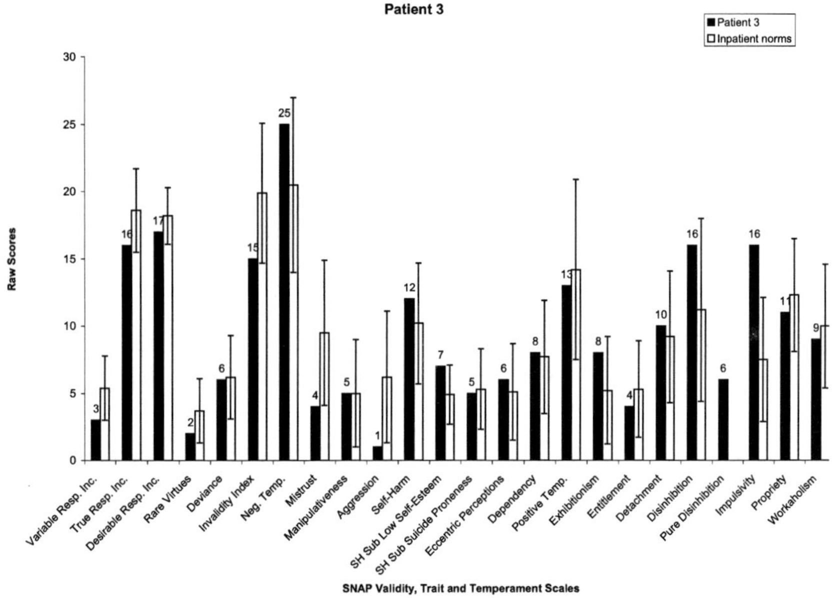

Figure 41. SNAP Temperament scales, comparison to inpatient norms

Within the temperament scales, in comparison to the normal population, the scales "Negative Temperament", "Self Harm" with subscales "Low Self Esteem" and "Suicide Proneness", and the scale "Impulsivity" are considered outside the norm (figure 40).Thus, compared to normal populations, the patient describes himself experiencing more negative emotions, tending to overreact to stresses of daily life, and endorsing more self-destructive thoughts and behaviors. In the scale "Disinhibition", the patient agrees to statements that say he does not show a lot of regard for the consequences of his behavior or endorses experiences without showing a lot of regard for social or legal norms or to potential risks. In the scale "Impulsivity", he agrees to statements like "I often act without thinking", or "I generally do not like to have detailed plans".

As can be seen in figure 41, this patient's raw scores lie within the norms of a clinical population described by Clark (1993), apart from two exceptions. As in the STIPO, he reports very little aggression (outside the norm) and reports significantly more impulsivity than inpatients. Similar to the comparison to a normal population, here the high scores in the scale "Negative Temperament" stand out as well.

The results in the scales "Negative Temperament", "Self-Harm", and "Impulsivity", especially the high T-Scores in comparison to a normal population, as well as the fact that most of his results can be found within the norms of a clinical sample, clearly indicate personality pathology; and according to Clark (1993) are especially strongly related to the DSM diagnoses Borderline, Antisocial, Histrionic Personality Disorder.

2.3.4.2 Diagnostic Scales

In the Diagnostic Scales (figure 42), with one interesting exception, the dimensional ratings of the personality disorders lie within the norm range of a male college student sample. Surprisingly, the patient does not reach a high dimensional score in narcissistic personality disorder, which his therapist and the team at the hospital had diagnosed, but in contrary, here he received his lowest dimensional score, falling outside of the norm range. It can be postulated that this patient might have denied endorsing any items indicating narcissistic pathology. This is affirmed when noting that his raw score of 4 is outside of the norm range of college students (mean 10.7; sd 4.0) as well as of inpatients (mean 8.5; sd 4.4) (Clark, 1993). Compared to the college sample, his highest dimensional scores, tipping toward the upper limit of the norm range, can be found in schizoid personality disorder, borderline personality disorder and avoidant personality disorder.

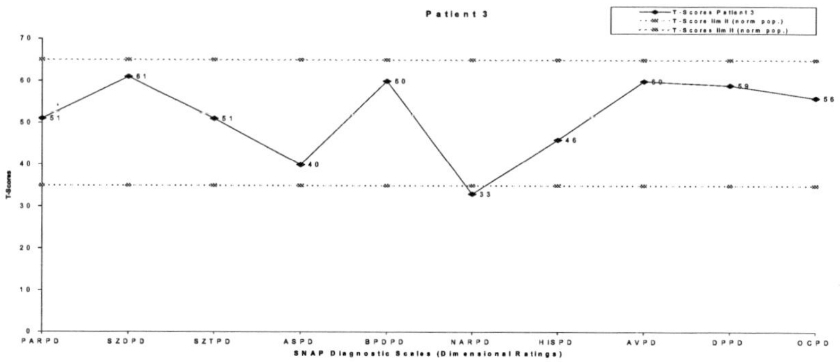

Figure 42. SNAP diagnostic scales (dimensional scores), comparison to norm T-Scores

Compared to the clinical sample (figure 43), he falls into the inpatient norms in all personality disorders but paranoid, antisocial and narcissistic personality disorders. Again, the question of denying these items (e.g. not endorsing "I deserve special recognition") can be posed. The highest score here is found in borderline personality disorder and obsessive-compulsive personality disorder. Overall, the high results in the diagnostic scales when compared to the normal sample, as well as the results mainly falling into the norms of an inpatient sample, can be interpreted as showing considerable amount of personality pathology, but still being in the healthier realm of inpatient populations.

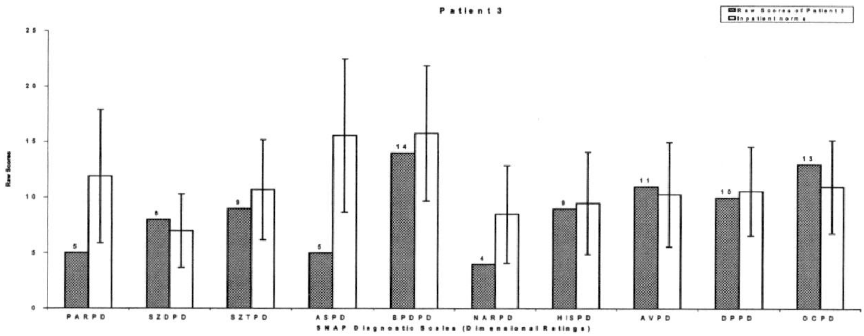

Figure 43. SNAP diagnostic scales (dimensional scores), comparison to inpatient norms

2.3.5 Results of IIP-PD

In the *Inventory of Interpersonal Problems Personality Disorders Scales (IIP-PD)* by Pilkonis et al. (1996) several topics were assessed: interpersonal sensitivity, interpersonal ambivalence, and aggression. This instrument is thought to be a good screening tool for the assessment of personality disorder versus no personality disorder. The patient reached an overall score of 1.07, slightly below the cut-off score of 1.1 (Stern et al., 2000), which differentiates between patients who clearly have a personality disorders versus the patients who do not. As it is very close to the threshold, it is apparent that this patient exhibits a rather high degree of personality pathology, illustrated by increased interpersonal sensitivity (e.g. “I feel attacked by other people too much”), high interpersonal ambivalence (e.g. “It is hard for me to do what another person wants me to do”) and elevated aggression (e.g. “I lose my temper too easily”), and confirms the impression gained so far.

2.3.6 Results of BFI-44

In the self-report measure *Big Five Inventory (BFI-44)* by John, Donahue & Kentle (1991), the patient’s personality was examined in terms of the Five-Factor-Model of Personality. Compared to norm values from a US-American sample consisting of 711 college students (Benet-Martinez & John, 1998), this patient’s level of “Extraversion”, his level of “Agreeableness” and his level of “Conscientiousness” are all in the normal range. His results in comparison to the norm sample are shown in figure 44.

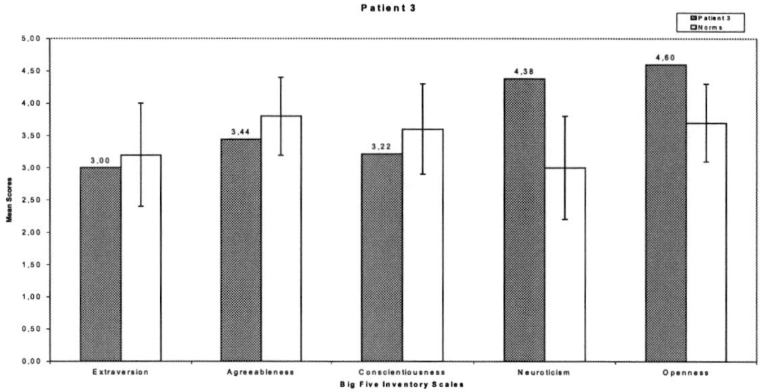

Figure 44. BFI-44 scales, comparison to college norms

Clearly, the level of "Neuroticism" and his level of "Openness for Experience" are outside the norm. High levels of "Neuroticism" are typical for personality disorders, especially BPD (Widiger & Costa, Jr., 1994) and are reflected, for example, in items like "is depressed", "can be tense", "can be moody". The high level of "Openness for Experience" fits to a person who is or sees her/himself as artistic and creative, as this factor assesses originality and curiosity, for example in items like "is inventive", "is curious about many different things" or "values artistic, aesthetic experiences".

2.3.7 Results of PANAS

The *Positive and Negative Affect Schedule (PANAS)* by Watson, Clark & Tellegen (Watson, Clark, & Tellegen, 1988) assesses the overall tendency for positive and negative affect as well as several mood scales like fear, hostility, joviality or serenity. The patient described the degree of experiencing different mood states during the last few weeks by use of a list of adjectives, for example words like "attentive", "fearless" or "angry".

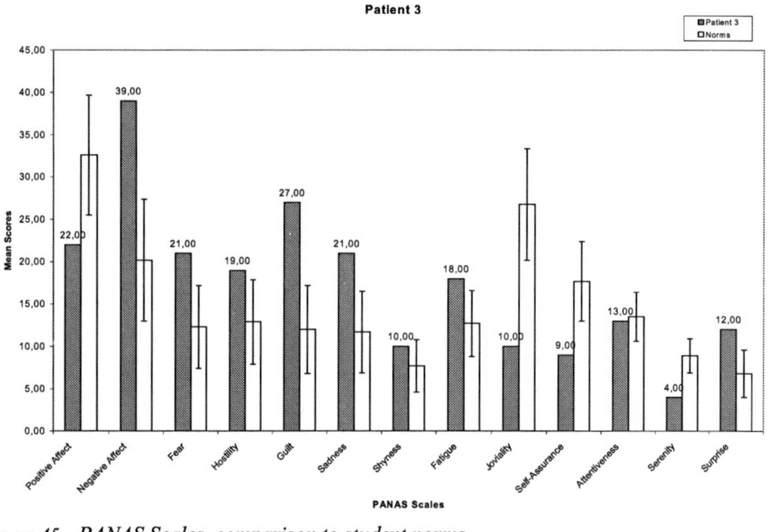

Figure 45. PANAS Scales, comparison to student norms

His results can be seen in figure 45 and indicate a strong tendency toward negative affect as well a very low score on the positive affect scale. Also in most of the negative affect subscales, namely in the scales "Fear", "Hostility",

“Guilt”, “Sadness”, he consistently described his mood states as outside of the norm, that is more negative than the norm. Accordingly, in most of the positive affect subscales “Joviality” and “Self-assurance” his scores were below the normal scores, indicating clearly less positive affect than the norm. Only in the subscale “Surprise” he presents himself above the norm, stating he experienced the states “amazed” or “astonished” more often than the norm.

2.3.8 <u>Results of Buss-Durkee-Inventory</u>

In the *Buss-Durkee-Inventory* (1957), the patient describes himself as employing a certain degree of hostility in his daily life. Although his scores are within in the norm range (compare figure 46), he did present high scores of different kinds of hostility; in particular his scores of “Suspicion”, “Resentment”, “Indirect hostility”, “Irritability”, and the “Total Irritability” score are slightly higher than in the norm sample of 85 male students (Buss & Durkee, 1957). He portrayed himself experiencing less guilt, verbal hostility and assault than the norm sample. Overall, this patient presented himself as moderately hostile, which matches the results in the other measures, in which he did not endorse aggressive or hostile items very much. This self-reported moderate levels of aggression do stand in certain contrast to the clinical impression, especially the “Aggression” domain in the STIPO.

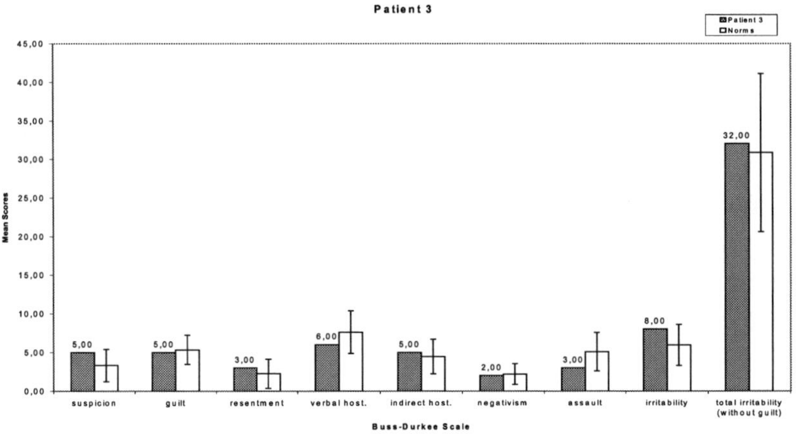

Figure 46. Buss-Durkee Inventory, comparison to student norms

2.3.9 Results of Brief Symptom Inventory

The *Brief Symptom Inventory* by Derogatis (1993) was used as a method to assess other symptoms of psychopathology and screen for other diagnoses. Again, it is of interest how many symptoms from DSM axis I diagnoses this patient, located at Borderline Personality Organization, would present. His results will be compared to the norms of a healthy sample and of an inpatient sample.

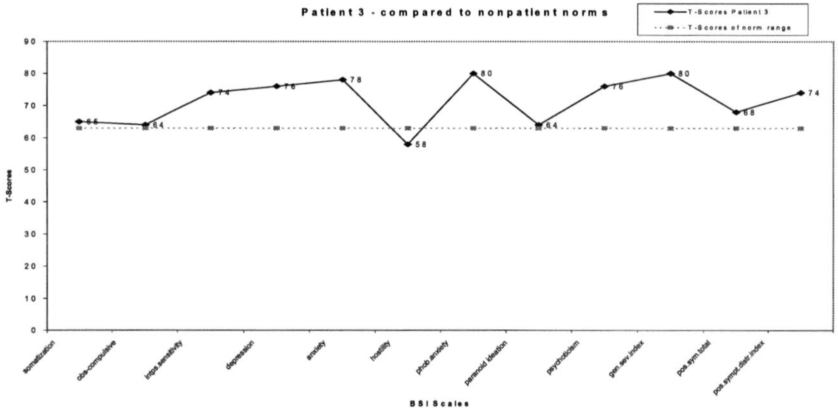

Figure 47. BSI scales, comparison to nonpatient norms

In comparison to the normal sample (figure 47) , his results clearly exceed the clinically relevant levels of T-scores of 63 in all but one case. Interestingly, only in the subscale "Hostility", he described less pathology than in the other scales, which matches his very benign self-description in the other instruments assessing different aspects of hostility or aggression. Contrary to this result, his scores in the rest of the scales, for example in "Somatization", "Obsessive-compulsiveness", "Depression", "Anxiety", "Paranoid ideation", "Phobic anxiety" or "Psychoticism" clearly exceeded the normal T-scores of the healthy sample. Compared to healthy individuals, he reported a lot of stress ("General Severity Index" T-score: 80) and described a large amount of symptoms ("Positive Symptom Total" T-score: 68) which he suffered from to a high degree ("Positive Symptom Distress Index" T-score: 74). In other words, this patient reported various symptoms from axis I diagnoses, as well as symptoms from areas that tap on axis II diagnoses (e.g. "interpersonal sensitivity"), but did not state experiencing an unusually high amount of hostility, as he did in the other instruments.

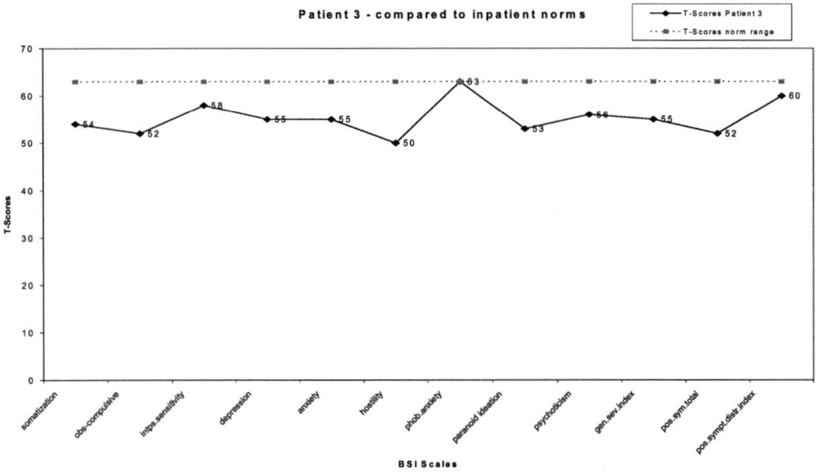

Figure 48. BSI scales, comparison to patient norms

In comparison to a clinical sample, his results more fit into the group of psychiatric inpatients. In figure 48, his results and the norm range based on an inpatient sample are presented. Here, his T-scores range between 50 and 63 and thus do not exceed the limit of the norm range. The highest score can be found in phobic anxiety, similar to the diagnosis of agoraphobia. The "General Severity Index" and "Positive Symptom Distress Index" do not reach a very high level when compared to a inpatient sample.

In total, the fact that this patient's profile matches an inpatient sample better than a sample of healthy individuals does confirm the need to diagnose and treat him as a rather disturbed patient. And as this screening instrument shows, he also presented a considerable degree of axis I pathology in addition to various interpersonal difficulties which had justified the classification in Borderline Personality Organization.

2.3.10 Summary Patient 3

In sum, this patient appeared as a higher level borderline patient (Borderline 1 as assessed with the STIPO) with narcissistic pathology, which primarily was assessed during the clinical STIPO interview. When inspecting his location among the clusters from hypothesis 1, he is part of cluster 1c, which can be considered a slightly less disturbed BPO subgroup. His high degree of identity diffusion was confirmed in the self-report measure IPO. Also, he presented himself with an extremely high amount of negative affect, complete lack of coping skills, strong self-destructive behavior, which he repeatedly demonstrated in several questionnaires (e.g. scores outside of the norm range in SNAP "Self-Harm", "Impulsivity", "Negative Temperament" Scales; "Negative Affect" Scale in PANAS; "Neuroticism" Scale in BFI-44). His problems in interpersonal relationships and representation of others, showing in levels of moderate pathology in the STIPO and IPO, also were assessed in a pathological score in the IIP-PD. An example of coinciding assessments in the STIPO and the self reports is the way the patient described his slightly impaired capacity for guilt. In the STIPO he reports that self-recriminative thoughts outweigh actions in trying to clear up the situation in which he has done something he knows is wrong. In the PANAS, for example, he states he has felt guilty and ashamed a lot recently, and therefore reaches a pathological score in the domain "guilt".

Overall, the key problems with this patient seem to be his rigid views of himself, difficulties in assessing others, strong impulsivity and self-destructive behavior.
It should be noted how the patient consistently did not endorse items that would describe him as hostile or aggressive, which showed in the IPO, the SNAP and the Buss-Durkee-Inventory or the BSI. An interesting aspect in the self-report assessments is that the patient reported more hostility in the Buss-Durkee inventory, which assesses hostility as a trait, whereas in the BSI, which focuses on the state (Shaw et al., 2003), he reported notably little hostility. A hypothesis could be that during the assessment, this could be a way of suppressing these feelings and impulses temporarily, perhaps in the sense of an inhibition of aggression, whereas in an assessment focusing on traits, a slightly different picture emerges.
The generally low hostility shown in the self-reports stands in stark contrast to the clinical impression in the STIPO and to the major reason for which he had been admitted to a psychiatric hospital, namely, a very aggressive, albeit self-directed, attack. So an open question in the assessment of this patient is that on the one hand, he presented himself rather stable and peaceful, figuratively like a friendly, slightly submissive boy scout; and on the other hand reported severely

aggressive outbursts, directed mainly against himself, but also against others. These contradicting sides and self-presentations are strong examples for the identity diffusion (especially STIPO domain "coherent sense of self") and difficulties when he gets in more intense contact with others. More thorough examination of how the patient suppresses this aggressive part of him and what makes him explode would be a focus of further assessment or therapy. One of the major goals of psychotherapy would be focusing on the identity diffusion and a stabilization of his life situation including a steady job and/or education. The recommendation would be to continue with Transference-Focused-Psychotherapy.

2.4. Example of a patient at Neurotic Personality Organization

2.4.1 Introduction and history

For comparison's sake, after three borderline patients of varying degree of pathology and at three different levels of BPO were described, now a high functioning patient with Neurotic Personality Organization (NPO) will be illustrated.

A 23 year-old single woman, who was born and had grown up in a European country and had come to a city in the US to study at a university two years ago, was interviewed in an outpatient setting. She had been recruited in the context of the study and was interested in participating.

She had no psychiatric history, no substance abuse history and was taking no psychiatric medication and had not been in psychotherapeutic treatment so far. She was interested in psychotherapy and mentioned she might consider starting psychoanalysis. She reported feeling depressed and anxious sometimes and had some difficulties in her relationships and thought psychotherapy might help her in dealing with these issues.

In her home country, she had grown up with her parents and two siblings and had gone to university for one year, and had come to a US-American city to get a university degree. She was living in student housing with friends. Her social network was rather diverse as she had friends in her home country with whom she kept in touch as well as a network of friends in the local city, most of whom were students as well. As she had received a stipend for her studies, she did not have to work to finance her education and presently was a full-time student. She

had had several romantic relationships in the past and presently was in a romantic relationship which she presented as rather serious.
The clinical impression she gave was that of an intelligent young woman who was quite ambitious with regard to her career and who interacted with me with a certain degree of shyness. She was very careful in answering the questions correctly and evoked the impression of taking every question very seriously.

2.4.2 Results of STIPO

The results in the STIPO will be explained in detail for each domain and subdomain separately. In the appendix the STIPO score form shows the individual items. Examples of the individual scores per item (on the 0-2 scale) within each domain will be mentioned in the text and explained. Also, the clinical judgment (on the 1-5 scale) will be provided. The results of this patient can be seen in both rating systems in figure 49, forming her profile. As mentioned above, the clinical judgment, rated on the 1-5 point scale, shown in the graph in the solid line, was used to compare the patient's results to the prototype and to establish her STIPO structural level. The "Impression based on scores", that is the mean scores per domain, consisting of the individual items per domain, is shown in the dotted line in the graph (transformed to a 1-5 scale) and was not used to compare the individual patient's results to the prototype. The discrepancies in the results of the 5-point ratings as opposed to the 3-point ratings (which had been transformed to a 5-point scale) are discussed in chapter 2.4.2.8.

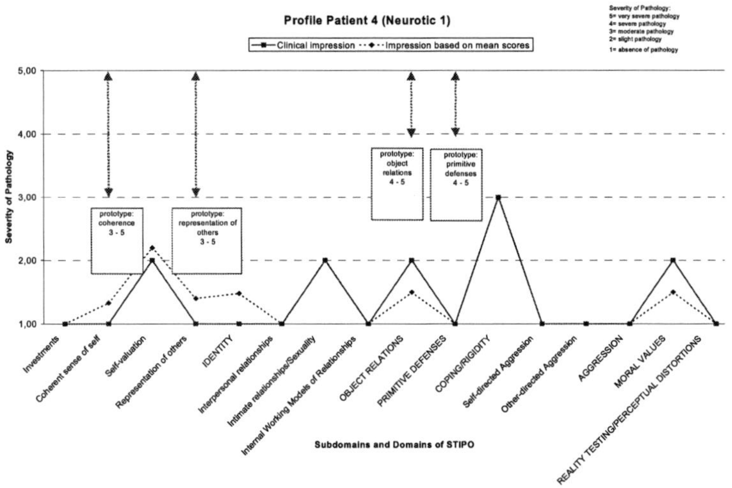

Figure 49. STIPO profile of patient 4 with domains of BPO prototype

2.4.2.1 Identity

In the first subdomain "Investments" of the overall domain "Identity", the patient reported that after school, she had gone to a university in her home country for an undergraduate degree, had worked for a year and then hat applied for a scholarship at a US university which she was granted. As she had only worked for a brief period of time and had primarily invested time into her education, the work section of the STIPO was skipped. She had been at this university in a master's program in an economic subject for two years and related that she was very successful and effective, meeting deadlines and getting A grades (score of 0 in "Studies-effectiveness"). She also reported having studied continuously, without any interruptions ("Stability":0), to enjoy her studies, although finding them quite challenging and labor-intensive, and that they did correspond to her professional goals of working in international commerce ("Enjoyment", "correspondence": 0). In her free time, she very lively described her investment in a literature and culture group, which met several times a week and which she had spent a lot of time with and to which she had given a lot of organizational input. As this activity was considered as serious investment in voluntary work, the items in this section were scored with "0". As an overall score in the subdomain "Investments" a "1" was given, taking into account her consistent and persistent investment into education and free time.

In the section "Coherence and continuity of the self", this patient was able to give a very profound self-description, illustrating an interesting contrast to the patients described earlier. She differentiated between positive and negative aspects of her personality, and showed the ability to connect both sides. For example, she said "I am a shy person, I am more introverted than others; but I am a good listener and am very interested in getting to know others; and I relate to different kinds of people; I value friendship and value to get to know others; I want more than one good friend; I am cheerful, if I am not worried". She also was able to elaborate further on the given aspects and overall, showed quite some reflection on her inner life (score of 0 in "Self-description"). She described having a continuous sense of herself across time (score of 0) and also in the present, for example feeling like the same person without any noticeable change when at school as opposed to with friends (score of 0 in "Consistent sense of self in present). Asked about taking on tastes and opinions, she did report to take into consideration other people's political or moral views when forming her point of view and also looking to the outside when trying to develop her taste in clothes or music (score of 1). In intimate relationships, she mentioned having difficulties holding on to her own views and tastes and tending to take on her boyfriend's tastes in order to make things easier, but also feeling to take these own as her own to a certain degree (1). In total, in spite of these two aspects in which she showed a tendency to adapt too much to others, a score of "1" was given, reflecting that this patient's self experience and life goals are coherent and continuous across time and situations.

In the domain "self valuation" this patient showed more insecurity and difficulties. She described comparing herself to a high degree to others and seeing her self-worth depend very much on these comparisons. She emphasized that these comparisons occurred especially with people from the more extraverted US culture, which she experienced very different from her more family-oriented European home country. She did illustrate this having a high impact on her self-worth (score of 2 in "Self valuation"). She expressed not feeling consistently superior to others (0 in "positive comparative self evaluation"), but feeling inferior to others in many situations, although having learnt to reassess the differences between her and others in many situations (score of 1 in "negative comparative self evaluation"). Her self-esteem did not fluctuate (score of 0), but she did describe other people's feedback influencing her sense of self-worth in a powerful way. She described this high impact being especially prominent in the academic field, conveying the impression of being rather competitive and success-oriented (score of 1 in "self-esteem external influence"). An overall score in the subdomain "self valuation" of "2" was chosen in order to reflect a somewhat realistic, but also somewhat negative, perhaps overly self-critical self-esteem.

In the subdomain "representations of others", this patient gave a slightly superficial description of her boyfriend as the most important person in her present life (score of 1). She portrayed him as an "overly kind, sincere, interested person; meaning well, is supportive, is interested in what you are saying, is patient". The description occurred to be slightly idealized, and upon request she could not think of any negative aspect and showed difficulties in providing a full and nuanced description of him. Regarding the question about the ability of getting a good understanding of other people's feelings and thoughts, she reported having no difficulties and hardly hurting other's feelings with her interpretations (score of 0). On the other hand, she acknowledged being unsure about what others thought about her and what they appreciated or disliked about her, implicating a rather low opinion about herself; she also mentioned being concerned rather much about other's opinions changing (score of 1 in "other's judgments"). When making up her mind about new people she met she did not report weighing in other's opinions very much ("external influence": 0). She also gave a very detailed, nuanced picture of her mother, describing her with sensitivity and empathy. For example, she described her as an intelligent woman with good conversational and social skills and a lot of life experience but also as someone having high expectations which weren't always easy to fulfill for her as daughter. As the description evoked a full and lively picture of her mother, a score of "0" was given. An overall score of "1" was chosen reflecting a stable and integrated sense of others. The decision to give a rating in the healthiest realm (instead of a score of 2) was made because the difficulties in describing her boyfriend are more likely to reflect difficulties in the area of object relations and romantic relationships as opposed to identity disturbances and will be given more weight in the next section.

In total, this patient illustrated a case of consolidated identity. The patient presented several typically neurotic difficulties like low self-worth and a sense of competitiveness or over-ambitiousness, but did not show identity instability per se and therefore a score of "1" was given.

2.4.2.2 Object Relations

In the subdomain "Interpersonal Relationships" of "Object Relations", this patient described several close friends she had known and kept in touch for many years. Due to her move to the USA, she could only keep in touch with her old friends from her home country via telephone but portrayed these friends as people with whom she shared even the more personal things. Also, she mentioned two friends she had gotten to know in the city with whom friendships were still evolving, but whom she trusted and felt they were open with her as well (score of 0 in "social isolation"). She reported no problems or fights with her close friends (0 in "problems/volatility") nor having difficulties when her friends were not available to her for any reason (0 in "response to stress"). The friendships she described had lasted from her childhood and she described being in touch continuously with her friends. Also, she denied having difficulties or fights with coworkers, fellow students, supervisors or teachers (score of 0 in "conflict at work/school". The quality of her friendships and the continuous and stable contact with several friends throughout the years, as well as the absence of conflicts in her friendships was rated with an overall "1".

In the subdomain "Intimate Relationships and Sexuality", the patient mentioned three relationships in the past five years of which she considered the present relationship as the most significant. She had been in a relationship with her partner in her home country for one year and after she left for the US, they broke up because the separation was very difficult for her to bear; then he followed to the US and the relationship continued. She described this relationship as a serious and supportive relationship, albeit not too stable in the past and gaining stability in the last months only. Besides the slightly unstable course of the relationship in the past, she talked about some difficulties which had a certain influence on the harmony of the relationship, for example different ideas of which priority was given to the relationship on his behalf. A score of "1" was given for the "history of relationships". Asked about the mutual trust and interdependence she confirmed he could depend on her but was unsure if she could depend on him, mentioning several phases in the relationship when he was not sure about their future and was not as open as she was, which had caused difficulties and raised the question of how much she could trust and rely on him and his feelings (score of 1 in "interdependency"). She also described herself as needing him more and investing more into the relationship, thus having the impression that she was giving more than he was. She remained unsure about this question, thus the question was scored with a "1" ("relationship economics"). The patient reported being sexually active within this relationship and being satisfied, and having had sexual encounters only within her relationships (0 in "sexual activity"), but reported being rather shy about sexuality and feeling inhibited frequently even in her long-lasting relationships (1 in "sexual inhibition"). She described enjoying the sensual aspects of sexuality and finding sexuality to intensify the emotional closeness she experienced with her partner (scores of 0 in "sensuality", "love and sex"). In total, this section was scored with a "2", taking into account the long-lasting relationship which was overall described as harmonious, but also weighing in the doubts she had regarding the mutuality of openness and interdependence as well as her slight sexual inhibition.

This patient reported no pathology in the subdomain "Internal Working Models of Relationships". Neither did she report having difficulties empathizing with others (score of 0), nor did she confirm experiencing disrespect or feeling disregarded frequently (scores of 0 in "Entitlement 1, 2"). She described herself as someone who respects other people's privacy (0 in "Autonomy of others") and repeated how much she valued friendship and made sure to keep in touch with her friends. Thus, all the items were scored with "0" and an overall score of "1" reflects that this patient did not regard her relationships in terms of need fulfillment and could experience empathy with and interest for others.

An overall score of "2" was chosen for the section "Object Relations". This patient presents a slightly neurotic pattern of well-functioning friendships, of durable and satisfying quality, but presenting a certain degree of impairment in her intimate relationships, especially in the sexual area. As she reported being somewhat inhibited sexually and having difficulties establishing a long-term and trusting relationship, these aspects are giving a certain weight in the overall rating. This is the only area where she tends to see her relationships more in terms of need fulfillment.

2.4.2.3 Primitive Defenses

This patient reported no use of primitive defenses. This is a very good example showing that this section clearly discriminates between neurotic and borderline patients. For example, she described being guarded in general and being careful in contact with others, but vividly described having several friendships with whom she could share everything without worrying at all (score of 0 in "paranoia"). This is a stark contrast to the borderline patients portrayed in the previous chapters. She denied using erratic behavior or idealizing and devaluing things or people. Also, she was surprised about the question of "externalization", arguing that of course she took on the responsibility for her actions (score of 0). In total, all of the items were scored with "0" and an overall score of "1" was chosen, reflecting that no primitive defenses were employed and if so, pathology would be expected in the area of higher level defenses, which was examined in the area "Coping and Rigidity".

2.4.2.4 Coping and Rigidity

In the domain of advanced defenses, "Coping and Rigidity", the patient was asked for a stressful event in the last five years and described the stressful exam period at her university. She said that during this time she was very tense and was under a lot of pressure. One of her strengths in times like this episode seemed to be her ability to anticipate, which she illustrated by describing how she was able to divide up her time in order to fulfill all her tasks (score of 0 in "anticipation"). But she did describe having difficulties suppressing distressing thoughts and admitted she tended to obsess over all the things she had to do to get through the situation (2 in "suppression"). Also, she portrayed herself as a person who does not respond very flexible to changes of plans (1 in "flexibility") and who tends to be very self-critical and perfectionistic up to the degree of impeding her performance through these very high expectations of herself (scores of 1 in "self-blame", "perfectionism"). She said she needed to hear from others how excessive her self-criticism was in order to stop it. In times of stress, as she reported, she often got overwhelmed and thus turned passive instead of proactive (score of 1): She also inclined to worry very much about things that might go wrong or might turn out complicated (2 in "worrying"). Asked about her general attitude towards challenges, she replied she only seeked out challenges if she "could live up to the challenge", describing

a somewhat avoidant outlook on things when the opportunities seemed difficult to assess (score of 1 in "challenge").
In total, it becomes clear that this is the weakest section for this patient. She portrayed herself as experiencing stress easily and feeling overwhelmed quickly. In difficult times, she seemed not to be able to use coping strategies or to adapt to demanding situations easily. The impression of a very ambitious person who demanded very much from herself was confirmed with these questions. An overall score of "3" was chosen in order to reflect her tendency to rigid coping.

2.4.2.5 *Aggression*

In the subdomain "Self-directed Aggression", this patient did not report any self-directed aggression. She had no suicidal history (score of 0 in "suicidality"), did not engage in risky behavior (score of 0) and had never cut or burnt her skin (score of 0 in "relief"). All of the items were scored with "0" and an overall rating of "1" was given.

Also in the subdomain of "Other-directed Aggression", she did not endorse any of the behaviors, denying loosing her temper or attacking or intimidating others. This confirmed her having a well integrated personality structure and all of the individual items were rated with 0 and an overall score of "1" was given.
In the overall rating of aggression a score of "1" takes into account that this patient does not direct anger or aggression toward herself or behave aggressively toward others. She described herself as someone who does not explode easily, instead tending to ruminate about things, getting critical with herself and perhaps being over-controlled. It becomes clear that her major difficulties lie in coping mechanisms which are linked with her high expectations and rather low self-esteem.

2.4.2.6 *Moral Values*

In the domain "Moral Values", this patient described following an internalized moral code when deciding upon right or wrong and rarely being tempted when confronted with immoral opportunities (scores of 0 in "internalized moral values"; "questionable opportunities"). She did admit lying occasionally about things that might make her look bad in front of others (1 in "lying/deceit"). At the same time, she described feeling very guilty about these lies and generally being very self-critical and guilt-ridden when doing something that might be considered not correct (1 in "guilt") . It became obvious that she had a slightly rigid way of holding on to her moral code and feeling anxious and blaming herself in interpersonal situations, for example avoiding confrontation with the other person when an excuse might be appropriate after having done something wrong, perhaps even being purposefully mean (1 in "sadism").

In total, a score of "2" was given in the domain "Moral Values". This rating takes into account that this patient showed no antisocial behavior and had a very strong sense of right and wrong but had difficulties in applying it to all of the situations in which it might be required, especially when other people are involved. Here she relates tending to engage in ruminative self-recrimination instead of proactive efforts to make amends. This could be considered to reflect a harsh superego, which appears especially in her self-critical thoughts and behaviors.

2.4.2.7 Reality Testing and Perceptual Distortions

With regard to "Reality Testing", this patient reported no perceptual distortions or disturbance in reality testing. In contrast, she gave the impression of being a very rational, controlled person who does not overreact nor become paranoid. She reported no dissociative episodes or depersonalization, in fact she was surprised by these questions as these experiences seemed very unfamiliar to her. The individual items were scored with "0" and an overall rating of "1" was given, confirming that these aspects, which are rather common with borderline patients, are unknown to this neurotic patient.

2.4.2.8 Comparison of Clinical impression versus item-based impression

With this patient, again the results of the 5-point ratings are rather close to the 3-point ratings. Slight discrepancies can be found for example in the "representation of others" (item based 1.4 versus clinical 1.0) and the overall "identity" score (1.5 versus 1.0), the former being caused by her elevated scores in the slightly idealized boyfriend description. The latter could be explained through the fact that the mean score takes in the elevated scores in the "self valuation" section as well. In the overall "Object Relations" score (1.5 versus 2.0) and the "Moral Values" score (1.5 versus 2.0) it is obvious that the clinical rating weighed in more pathology than the mean scores. However, the discrepancies are not very large, indicating a strong overlap between item-based and clinical ratings.

2.4.2.9 Fulfillment of prototypical criteria

This patient fulfilled none of the four prototypical criteria. In the domain "Coherent sense of self" the patient was scored with a "1", showing the absence of identity diffusion, and clearly not fulfilling the necessary pathology for the prototype. This patient's score of "1" in "representation of others" is also clearly not within the prototypical realm of scores between 3 and 5 and shows that there are no great difficulties in understanding and assessing others and in the perception of others' view of the subject. Also in this area, she clearly does not fulfill the prototype. In the overall domain of "Object Relations", her score of "2" indicates the presence of strong and durable attachments with some difficulties in romantic relationships. The score does not fulfill the necessary level of pathology for the prototype, which is a score of "4" or higher. In "Primitive Defenses", in which a score of "4" or higher is the prototypical level of pathology, this patient was rated with a "1", reflecting that primitive defenses are not endorsed. Again, here she does not fulfill the prototype. In total, none of the prototypic criteria are fulfilled, clearly showing that this patient is in the neurotic realm and fits well into group 3 of the examined sample: this is the healthiest, high level group of patients with neurotic personality organization (NPO), whose difficulties do not lie in the areas of the BPO prototype, but in others, for example in self-valuation, sexuality or coping abilities.

2.4.3 Results of IPO

In the *Inventory of Personality Organization (IPO)* by Clarkin, Foelsch, and Kernberg (2001), this patient's scores were rather close to the STIPO scores, but in most of the cases the IPO score was slightly above the clinical score in the STIPO's corresponding domain. Her level of identity diffusion in the IPO lay at a mean score of 1.5 and rather close to the STIPO score of 1.00, indicating a rather high overlap in self-description and clinical judgment and confirming the similar content of the two instruments. The slightly elevated IPO score again could be explained with the fact that the items assessing self-valuation (which is one of the more pathological areas with this patient) also are part of the mean "Identity" score. In "Primitive Defenses" (IPO mean score 1.5 versus STIPO

mean score 1.00), in "Aggression" (IPO mean score 1.2 versus STIPO score 1.0) and in "Reality Testing" (IPO mean score 1.6 versus STIPO score 1.00) the self-reported level of pathology and the clinical rating are rather close to each other. The fact that the self-reported score is slightly higher in these domains could be explained through the scoring procedure: Clinically, for this patient a score of "1" (absence of pathology) or "2" (slight pathology) was considered, and in these cases, the lower level of pathology was chosen. In contrast, the self-reported score is the mean score of many items, thus resulting in a "finer" score.
At last, in the domain "Moral Values", the IPO score (1.7) is slightly lower than the STIPO score (2.0), which in this case could be explained with the choice of the more pathological score of "2" in the STIPO, whereas the IPO result again is the "finer" score.
In total, the IPO results in the primary scales "Identity", "Primitive Defenses" and "Reality Testing" and in the secondary scale "Aggression" correspond to a high degree to the STIPO clinical ratings in these scales, but are slightly higher than the STIPO ratings, whereas the results of the IPO Secondary Scale "Moral Values" is slightly lower than the STIPO rating, perhaps due to the more categorical decision made in the clinical STIPO rating as opposed to the more dimensional mean score in the IPO.

2.4.4 Results of SNAP

A large and diverse amount of information regarding this patient's temperament characteristics and personality pathology can be obtained from the *Schedule for Nonadaptive and Adaptive Personality (SNAP)* by Clark (1993), so it will be looked at more in depth. First, we can examine the patient's Temperament Scales in comparison to the unisex norms of a norm sample of 561 normal adults (Clark et al., in press). Then, we can compare her Temperament scales to a unisex sample of 143 inpatients (Clark et al., in press). With regard to the diagnostic scales, we will compare her dimensional personality disorder ratings to the norms of a sample of 345 female college students and to the unisex norms of a sample of 45 inpatients (Clark, 1993).

2.4.4.1 Validity, Trait and Temperament Scales

For this patient, the question is different than with the previous three patients. As we consider this patient a neurotic patient, we want to compare her results to healthy individuals and to inpatients, expecting her results to resemble those of the healthy individuals more. Also, we will examine where her results fall in relation to inpatients.

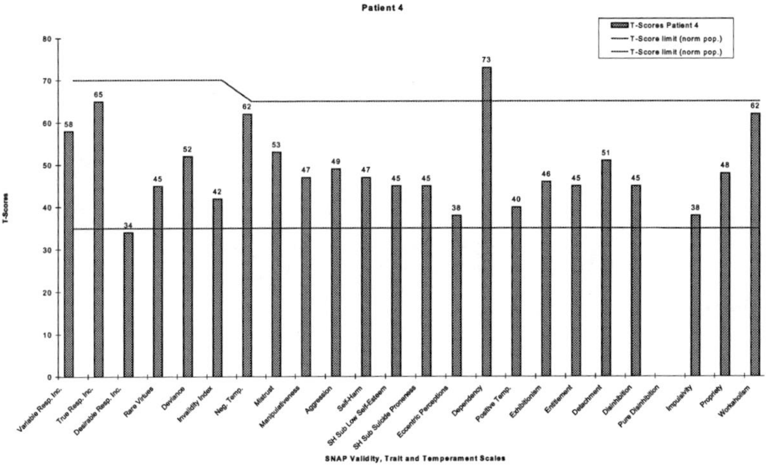

Figure 50. SNAP Temperament scales, comparison to norm T-Scores

In figure 50, we can see that in all but one of the validity, trait and temperament scales, her T-Scores, which were calculated based on a college sample, lie within the norm range of healthy individuals. “Normal” t-scores range from 35 to 70 in the validity scales and from 35 to 65 in the temperament and trait scales. They are indicated by the two lines in the figure. T-scores outside of this range are considered unusual.

Compared to a normal population, all of the results in the validity scales fall into the normal range, only the “desirable response inconsistency” is just below the norm range. This result shows that this patient does not tend to reply in a socially desired way. A similar result can be found in the validity scales when compared to inpatients (figure 51). The results are within the norm range of the inpatient sample, most significantly the “Invalidity Index” is clearly lower than the inpatients’ range, implying a less invalid response style than seen in the inpatient sample. Thus, this patient's response patterns do not suggest invalidity, both compared to normal individuals and to inpatients.

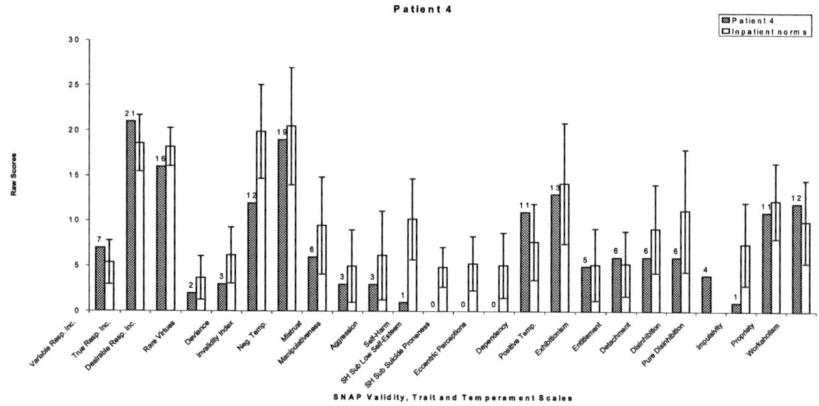

Figure 51. SNAP Temperament scales, comparison to inpatient norms

Within the temperament scales, in comparison to the normal population, all of the scales are in the norm range, the only scale clearly standing out is " Dependency" (figure 50). Thus, compared to normal populations, the patient described herself as looking for external advice and approval for her actions and decisions and feeling hesitant when she had no one to depend on. For example, she endorsed items like "I base many of my decisions on what other people think". The other elevated score, but still within the norm limits, can be seen in "Workaholism". Apart from these results, she depicted her personality in line with the norms of a normal student sample.

As figure 51 shows, many of this patient's raw scores lie at the lower end or outside of the norms of a clinical population described by Clark (1993). Especially in the scales in which the BPO patients described earlier achieved high scores, for example in self-harm or impulsivity, this patient achieves a negligible score. The only scales worthwhile mentioning are, same as in the comparison to healthy individuals, her scores in "Dependency" and in "Workaholism", which are higher than the inpatient mean, albeit within the inpatient norm range. The high score in dependency confirms the impression she gave in the "Intimate Relationship" Domain of the STIPO, that is clinging to her boyfriend to a certain degree and having difficulties being on her own without him. The high score in workaholism matches the very ambitious, perfectionist impression she gave in the STIPO. In total, the results in the trait and temperament scales being within the range of a normal population and at the lower end or outside of the range of a clinical sample, reinforce the impression of a neurotic patient with no borderline personality pathology, who showed some dependent and work-oriented traits.

2.4.4.2 Diagnostic Scales

Compared to a female college student sample, in the diagnostic scales (figure 52) none of the scores are outside of the norm range in the dimensional ratings of the personality disorders. The highest dimensional scores, tipping at the upper end of the range, can be seen in obsessive compulsive personality disorder, avoidant personality disorder, and dependent personality disorder. The lowest score can be found in antisocial personality disorder. This profile corresponds to the clinical impression this patient evoked in the STIPO. She clearly does not endorse any antisocial or borderline traits – in contrast to the previous patients – but her deficits can be found in the traits corresponding to the higher level personality disorders. Her dependent attitude, achievement- oriented thinking and perfectionism might be moving her closer to the neurotic end of the personality disorders (compare figure 1 in chapter II 2). When examining the dimensional scores of dependent personality disorder across the different patient groups (more details in section V.1.), it is interesting to note that this patient is the only outlier in the cluster of neurotic patients. This indicates her dependent attitude moving her closer to the diagnosis of a dependent personality disorder than the other patients from this group.

When regarding these traits as they are part of the DSM diagnoses and are assessed with the diagnostic scales, now we can examine where her results fall in comparison to the clinical sample (figure 53). In fact, in these Cluster A diagnoses (obsessive-compulsive personality disorder, avoidant personality disorder, dependent personality disorder), she achieved the highest scores, including scores which are even slightly above the inpatient mean. Again, in contrast to the previous patients, her results in the antisocial or borderline dimensional ratings are very low. Overall, it can be doubted that this patient would fulfill the diagnostic criteria for a proper personality disorder, for example in a clinical interview assessing these personality disorders, but it is noteworthy that she has several rigid aspects of her personality which definitely move her toward the neurotic end of the spectrum of personality disorders. The impression gained in the STIPO is confirmed in that respect, as she is a neurotic patient whose difficulties lie in the area of intimate relationships and also in over-ambitiousness, need for control and slight rigidity in the field of work.

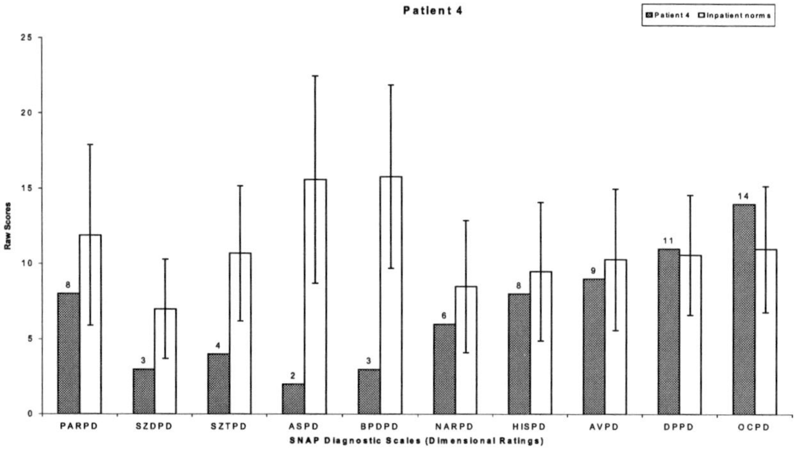

Figure 52. SNAP diagnostic scales (dimensional scores), comparison to norm T-Scores

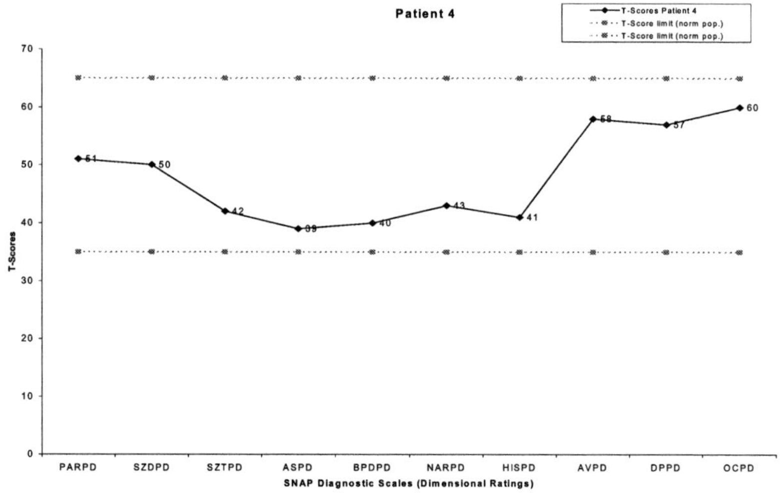

Figure 53. SNAP diagnostic scales (dimensional scores), comparison to inpatient norms

2.4.5 ***Results of IIP-PD***

In the *Inventory of Interpersonal Problems Personality Disorders Scales (IIP-PD)* by Pilkonis et al. (1996) several topics were assessed: interpersonal sensitivity, interpersonal ambivalence, and aggression. This instrument is thought to be a good screening tool for the assessment of personality disorder versus no personality disorder. The patient reached an overall score of 0.93 which is clearly below the cut-off score of 1.1 (Stern et al., 2000) which differentiates between patients who clearly have a personality disorders versus the patients who do not. The low score confirms that this patient did not show a significant level of personality pathology. She did not endorse items to a high degree which assessed increased interpersonal sensitivity (e.g. "I feel attacked by other people too much"), high interpersonal ambivalence (e.g. "It is hard for me to do what another person wants me to do") or elevated aggression (e.g. "I lose my temper too easily"), and confirms that this patient does not have serious difficulties in interpersonal relationships.

2.4.6 ***Results of BFI-44***

In the self-report measure *Big Five Inventory (BFI-44)* by John, Donahue & Kentle (1991), the patient's personality was examined in terms of the Five-Factor-Model of Personality. Compared to norm values from a US-American sample consisting of 711 college students (Benet-Martinez & John, 1998), this patient's level of "Extraversion" is slightly below the norm range, whereas she described a level of "Neuroticism" slightly above the norm. The results in the remaining three scales "Agreeableness", "Conscientiousness" and "Openness" are within the normal range. Her results in comparison to the norm sample are shown in figure 54.

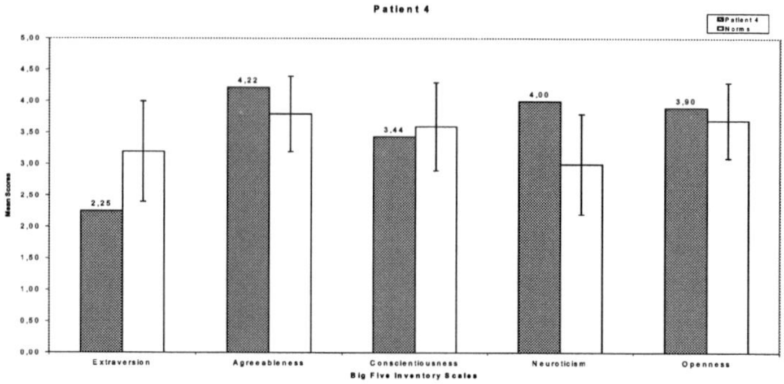

Figure 54. BFI-44, comparison to student norms

The low level of "Extraversion" indicates that this patient sees herself as someone who is not very outgoing, enthusiastic or talkative and matches the self-description of being rather shy and needing time to get to know others as she mentioned in the STIPO. It is interesting that her level of "Neuroticism" is outside of the norm, which is unusually high for a neurotic patient, and is rather close to the results of the Borderline patients described earlier. It is assessed through items like "is depressed", "can be tense", "can be moody" and thus leads to the conclusion that this scale might not differentiate as well between patients with BPO or NPO. Her high level of "Agreeableness" (within the norm range of the college sample) is in line with the findings in the previous self-reports, as this scale is comprised by items like "is considerate and kind to almost everyone" or "likes to cooperate with others". This matches her interest in others and the friendships described in the STIPO and to a certain degree, her dependent features in the SNAP. This high level of Agreeableness stands in stark contrast to the results of the Borderline patients. Her levels of "Conscientiousness" and "Openness" are elevated, but within the norm range. In total, these results coincide with the previous results, although the high level of "Neuroticism" is an interesting finding, especially when compared to the borderline patients.

2.4.7 ***<u>Results of PANAS</u>***

The *Positive and Negative Affect Schedule (PANAS)* by Watson, Clark & Tellegen (1988) assessed the overall tendency for positive and negative affect as well as several mood scales like fear, hostility, joviality or serenity. The degree of experiencing different mood states during the last few weeks was assessed by use of a list of adjectives, for example words like “attentive”, “fearless” or “angry”. The patient’s results can be seen in figure 55, where they are compared to 2076 college students (Watson, Clark, & Harkness, 1994):

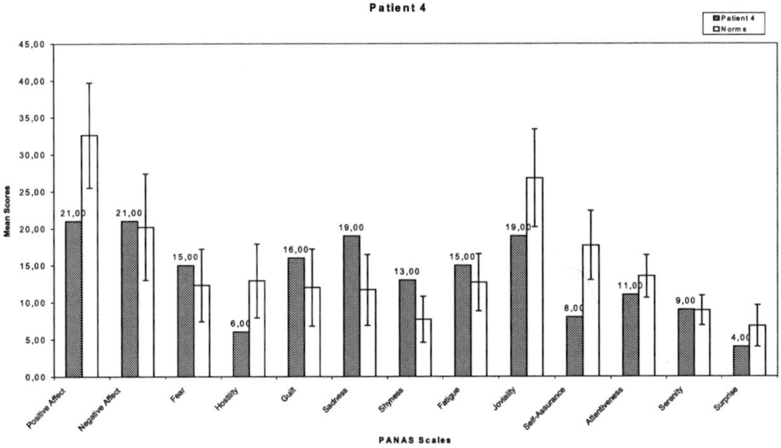

Figure 55. PANAS scales, comparison to student norms

The results indicate a slight tendency toward negative affect and a rather low score in positive affect. In the subscales assessing negative mood aspects she portrays herself as experiencing a high amount of “Sadness” and very little “Joviality”, as her results in these scales are outside the norm. Also her levels of “Shyness” and “Self-assurance” are outside the norm. As an interesting contrast to the borderline patients, whose levels of negative affect and hostility clearly exceeded the norm, she describes an average level of “Negative affect” and a very low level of “Hostility”.

Overall, these results are in line with the results in the other instruments, especially with the impression she evoked in the STIPO, having self-esteem difficulties and feeling very concerned about herself; as well with the low self esteem described in the SNAP, and with a higher level of “Negative Temperament” in the SNAP and “Neuroticism” in the BFI. The important difference to the BPO patients can be seen in the fact that this patient achieved a very low score in the borderline-typical scale of hostility and in the fact that her results in the negative temperament scales are not as extremely elevated as the other patients'.

2.4.8 Results of Buss-Durkee-Inventory

In the *Buss-Durkee-Inventory* (1957), this patient reached a very low level of irritability when compared to a sample of 74 female students (Buss & Durkee, 1957). The results are presented in figure 56. Her total irritability score is clearly lower than the norm range, also her scores in resentment, indirect hostility and negativism. Interestingly, her level of verbal hostility is rather high, although still within the norm range of the student sample, and the levels of indirect hostility and a negativistic attitude instead are low. This is the opposite pattern to the previously described borderline patients, who reported using more indirect hostility, negativism and suspicion. The high score in guilt corresponds to her STIPO-based impression of being very self-critical and hard on herself. In total, this patient described herself as person with very low levels of irritability, which is shown to others directly, if at all.

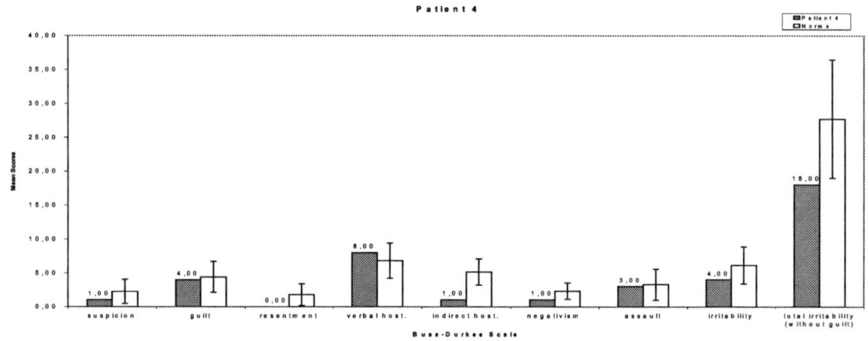

Figure 56. Buss-Durkee-Inventory, comparison to student norms

2.4.9 Results of Brief Symptom Inventory

The *Brief Symptom Inventory* by Derogatis (1993) was used as a method to assess other symptoms of psychopathology and screen for other diagnoses. The focus of evaluation is different for this patient. With patients 1 to 3, the question of comorbid axis I diagnoses in addition to the personality disorders was tested. Regarding this patient who is located at Neurotic Personality Organization it is interesting to assess if any axis I diagnosis might be predominant in her difficulties. Again, we can compare the patient to a healthy sample and to inpatient norms.

In comparison to the normal sample, only a few of her results, shown in figure 57, exceed the clinically relevant levels of T-scores of 63. In the subscales "Obsessive-compulsive", "Interpersonal Sensitivity" and "Depression", her scores are above the cut-off. In the other scales, for example in "Hostility", "Phobic Anxiety" and "Paranoid Ideation", her scores are clearly below the cut-off of normal T-scores of the healthy sample. The highest scores in "Interpersonal Sensitivity" and "Depression", assessed with "feelings of low self-worth", "feeling self-conscious with others" or "feeling blue", "feeling lonely", correspond to the traits this patient presented in the other instrument, that is self-worth problems and depressive tendencies. The high level in the obsessive-compulsive dimension, assessed for example through items like "having to double check what you do", is also not surprising as this was confirmed in several of the instruments (STIPO, SNAP). Again, the contrast to the Borderline patients is of interest, as this patient scores very low in the dimensions "Hostility" and "Paranoid Ideation", which were endorsed highly by all of the BPO patients. Compared to healthy individuals, she described experiencing an endurable amount of stress ("General Severity Index" T-score: 62), described not having a large number of symptoms ("Positive Symptom Total" T-score: 58), and reported suffering from these only to a certain degree ("Positive Symptom Distress Index" T-score: 65; just above the cut-off). In other words, this patient described only few symptoms from axis I diagnoses, for example a depressive and obsessive-compulsive tendency, and reported not to suffer from these very much.

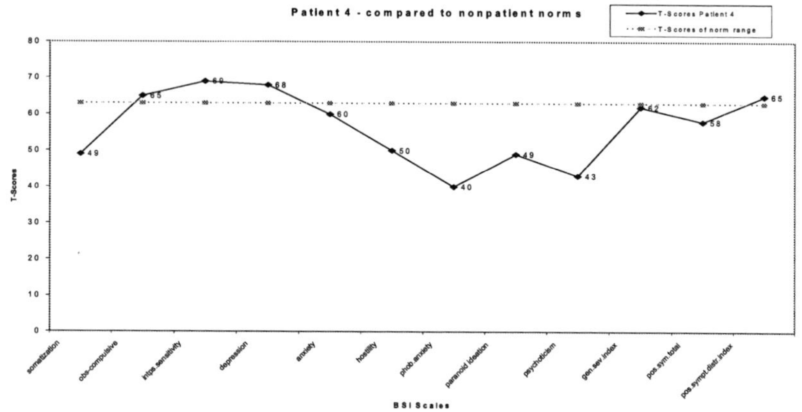

Figure 57. BSI scales, comparison to nonpatient norms

In comparison to a clinical sample (compare figure 58), her results clearly are different form the group of psychiatric inpatients. Here, her T-scores range between 34 and 55, thus are well below the limit of the norm range and do not fulfill the criteria for a "clinical case" as is defined in the manual by Derogatis (1993). The highest scores again can be found in "Obsessive-compulsive", "Interpersonal Sensitivity" and "Depression", emphasizing that these are her biggest difficulties. The "General Severity Index" and "Positive Symptom Distress Index" do not reach a high level at all when compared to an inpatient sample.

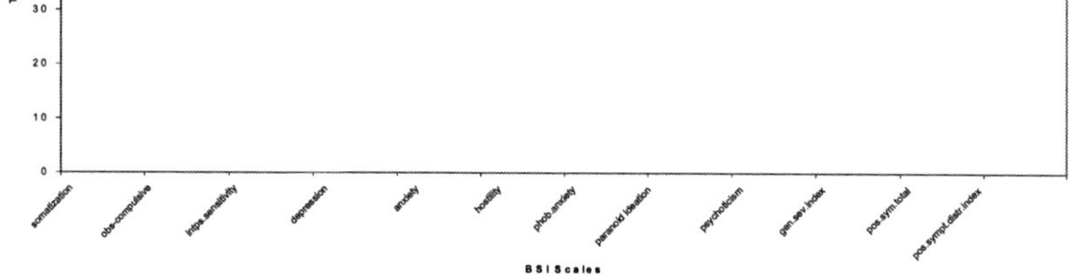

Figure 58. BSI scale, comparison to patient norms

In total, the fact that this patient's profile is very close to the sample of healthy individuals and does not match the inpatients at all does confirm that this patient definitely is not a severely disturbed patient located in BPO but is a patient whose difficulties lie primarily in neurotic problems like depression and obsessive-compulsiveness. These difficulties show differences to the other patients and imply that she should be diagnosed and treated according to a diagnosis of NPO.

2.4.10 __Summary Patient 4__

This patient was described in order to show the different levels of personality organization with corresponding foci of difficulties and subsequent treatment implications. In sum, this patient clearly is a neurotic patient (Neurotic 1 as assessed with the STIPO) whose primary difficulties lie in low self-worth, a tendency of being very self-demanding and in a certain level of depression. Regarding the clusters as emerged under hypothesis 1, she can be found in the third cluster; the healthiest, neurotic cluster. In the clinical STIPO interview the borderline typical deficits were not found, that is no identity diffusion, disturbed representation of others, strong impairment of object relations or use of primitive defenses. Moreover, in the STIPO a self-worth conflict was assessed as well as self-demanding and very ambitious traits, and difficulties in her intimate relationships. In IPO and IIP-PD, the absence of strong personality pathology was confirmed. The difficulties with intimate relationships and autonomy are suggested by an elevated score of the SNAP subscale dependency. The high demands this patient poses on herself were confirmed in the SNAP subscale "Workaholism" and the BSI dimension "obsessive-compulsiveness". In several of the self-report instruments, for example the SNAP subscales "Negative Temperament", the BFI Scale "Neuroticism", the PANAS Scales "Negative Affect", "Sadness" and "Guilt", as well as in the BSI dimension "depression", a tendency toward negative affect or depression was confirmed. It would be interesting to round out the existing information with a clinical interview assessing clinical diagnoses like mood disorders – it could be expected that this patient would fulfill the diagnostic criteria of a depressive disorder.

Overall, it becomes clear that the difficulties this patient suffers from are quite different from the deficits of the three Borderline patients described earlier. One of the essential conclusions is that this patient has a better perception, understanding and differentiation of mental states in self and others, which is referred to by Bateman and Fonagy as "mentalization" (Bateman & Fonagy, 2004a), and is shown here, for example, in the absence of strong difficulties in "representation of others" assessed with the STIPO. The ability to mentalize is an important element when deciding on the appropriate treatment, especially when taking into consideration insight-oriented treatments like psychoanalytic psychotherapy or psychoanalysis. For the decision over these forms of treatment a certain level of mentalization is necessary and is one of the foci of therapy, for example with Transference-Focused Psychotherapy (TFP; Clarkin, Yeomans & Kernberg, 1999; 2006). Severe difficulties with mentalization can be considered a counterindication for psychoanalysis. The implication of the thorough assessment with this patient is that she would be well suited for psychoanalytic treatment in which the main intrapsychic conflicts that are impeding her well-being and relationships could be worked through.

2.5. Comparison of the four single cases

Four patients were chosen to exemplify different levels of personality organization and to demonstrate the use of the STIPO as well its overlap and discrepancies to other diagnostic instruments. Also, it was shown how the STIPO based prototype of BPO differentiates between these patient groups.

Patient 1 was located at a low level of BPO (Borderline 2 as assessed with the STIPO), fulfilled all of the prototypical criteria and could be considered a typical Borderline patient. Throughout the instruments, she showed a lot of personality pathology, especially problems with impulsivity, aggression and dependency. Patient 2 (Borderline 3 in the STIPO) is a severely disturbed patient clearly fulfilling the necessary pathology in the STIPO and showing strong antisocial traits, extremely disturbed object relations, substance abuse problems and a parasitic life style. Patient 3 (Borderline 1 in the STIPO) is a higher level Borderline patient with narcissistic features, who fulfilled only two of the four prototypic criteria, namely identity difficulties, but was supported by valued object relations, and presented a mixed pattern of using primitive defenses. With this patient, the question of an inhibition of aggression is raised. Patient 4 is a neurotic patient (Neurotic 1 in the STIPO) whose problems differ from the other three patient and who does not show significant amounts of pathology in any of the BPO prototypical dimensions. Her deficits lie in the area

of self-worth, depression and a self demanding, slightly overambitious personality style. Again, this should emphasize the different levels of personality organization and make clear how the BPO prototype helps in easily identifying where a patient might be located.
When examining where these four patients fall in regard to the three clusters which emerged from the cluster analysis (hypothesis 1), patients 1 and 2 are part of cluster 1 (subgroup 1a), which is the most disturbed BPO group. Patient 3 is also located in cluster 1, but in the healthier subgroup 1c, considered as less disturbed and slightly less prototypical group. Finally, patient 4 is part of cluster 3, the NPO cluster. Hence, these four patients exemplify the use of the prototype in discriminating between different patient groups.

The instruments examining personality pathology or borderline-typical traits like the IIP-PD, the IPO, the SNAP or the Buss-Durkee Scale showed that the patients' assessment in the STIPO corresponded to a large degree to the self-reported deficits. Very generally stated, the level of pathology declined according to the personality organization location, that is patient 2 showing the most pathology, followed by patient 1, patient 3 and finally patient 4. For example, regarding the levels of total irritability in the Buss-Durkee-Scale, patient 2 reached a mean score of 58, patient 1 a mean score of 38, patient 3 reached a score of 32 and patient 4 a score of 18 (compare figure 59).

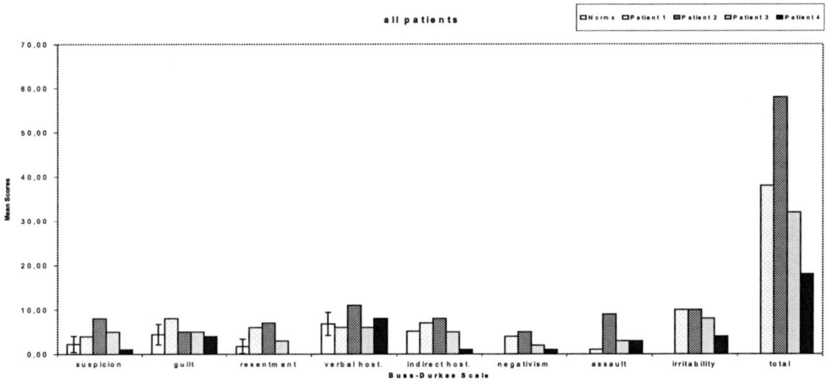

Figure 59. Buss-Durkee-Scale: compared across the four patients

Also, the ratings of the four patients in the prototypical domains of the STIPO are shown in figure 59 for comparison. Note that, for example in the fourth prototypical domain, Primitive Defenses, the ratings of the four patients, located on four different levels of personality organization, lie according to the levels of pathology: Patient 1, the most disturbed (BP3) , reached a score of 5, patient 2 located on BP2, was scored with a 4, patient 3 (BP1) with a 3 and the healthiest patient 4 (NP1) reached a score of 1. The vertical arrows indicate the range of prototypicality per domain. A figure with the complete profile, i.e. all of the STIPO domains, of the four patients is also shown in the appendix in figure 60.

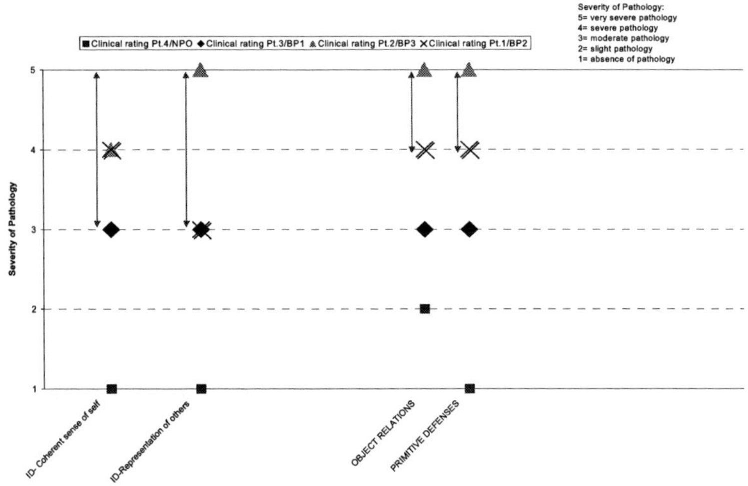

Figure 60. STIPO: the four prototypical domains compared across the four patients

The choice of possible treatments and prognosis depends on different aspects. The general life situation including working situation and relationship status ("work and love"), the level of personality organization, the capacity of gaining insight, as well as other factors like the consciousness of failure, concern about the future, ignorance about the situation, the presence of antisocial traits, as well as the motivation should be taken into consideration.

Patient 1 was in a steady situation regarding her studies and in a firm, albeit not very healthy, relationship. The stable work situation is a good precondition for therapy, as well as a certain amount of motivation to participate in treatment. On the one hand this patient was located on a lower level of personality organization, accompanied by some difficulties in insight and understanding mental states in self and others. On the other hand, she showed interest and a certain concern about her situation as well as no severe antisocial traits. In sum, this gives hope for being able to improve her situation with an insight-oriented treatment like TFP.

In contrast, patient 2 provided nearly no resources which could be used for a successful therapeutic relationship and potential change. She was located at the most disturbed level of personality organization, had been living off welfare for a long time and was not interested in working nor concerned about her present situation or future. She was not able to experience guilt, showed severe levels of aggression and hostility and a large array of antisocial traits. She did not evoke the impression of wanting to change nor gain insight into what caused her life situation. Outpatient treatment is not likely to help this patient, so extended inpatient treatment specialized on delinquent patients might be considered the choice.

Patient 3 was not involved in steady work or education, which would be an important precondition for therapy. Not being in a steady relationship but having some important attachments and being located at a higher level of BPO, is favorable for treatment success and prognosis. His capacity for insight is impoverished and he did not show a large degree of concern about his future, but was motivated to participate in treatment and showed no severe antisocial behaviors. Taking in these aspects, the recommendation would be to emphasize the importance of a more stable life situation to him and to continue working with him with TFP.

At last, patient 4 had the most favorable perspective, taken into consideration her being located in the neurotic realm, being in a steady relationship (which nevertheless would be one of the foci of therapy due to some relationship difficulties) and being very invested in her education. Also, she demonstrated a high interest in mental states of self and others, absence of antisocial traits, was concerned about herself and her important others, and showed readiness to work on her difficulties. In her case, psychoanalytic psychotherapy or psychoanalysis would be indicated.

VI DISCUSSION

This study describes how a theory-based prototype of Borderline Personality Organization derived from expert consensus and based on domains of the "Structured Interview of Personality Organization" (STIPO) was developed and examined empirically in a clinical sample. Using the expert consensus prototype of BPO as a basis, a variable describing each individual's similarity to the prototype was computed, i.e. a BPO similarity index. The BPO prototype, which operationalizes Kernberg's diagnostic system for personality disorder, was shown to differentiate between clinical groups and demonstrated good interrater-reliability, as well as convergent and incremental validity in predicting measures of axis II pathology. The usefulness of this prototype approach for the diagnosis of personality pathology and for deriving treatment implications and prognostic statements will be discussed.

1 Interpretation of the findings

1.1. Clinical groups (Hypothesis 1)

One of the main results of this study is the finding that the BPO prototype was able to discriminate between different clinical groups. Dimensional ratings of the four clinical STIPO scales employed to calculate the prototype were used to divide the sample into three clusters. These groups were significantly different with regard to general functioning, axis I symptoms, axis II symptoms and variables closely linked to axis II pathology.

The BPO group

As shown within the results of hypothesis 1, the first cluster could be interpreted as a group of patients located at the level of Borderline Personality Organization, with severe deficits in general functioning, showing significant levels of axis I pathology such as anxiety or depression, high scores in the SNAP diagnostic personality scales and high levels of negative affect, aggression, and other correlates of axis II. The patients in this group also presented high levels of identity diffusion and primitive defenses, in line with Kernberg's model (1984). This group was significantly different from the two other groups, a so-called "intermediate group" and a "neurotic group".

The intermediate group

The intermediate and neurotic groups demonstrated nearly no statistically significant differences between each other on most of the scales (assessing general functioning, axis I and axis II pathology), albeit one scale differentiated the intermediate from the neurotic group. The SNAP subscale “Self-Harm” seemed to make a distinction between the intermediate patients who appeared similar to the neurotic group in other variables, from this healthiest NPO group. Thus, finding an intermediate group is of particular clinical interest. If not for these findings, it would be tempting to condense the intermediate and neurotic group into a “less disturbed, higher level” group of patients.

On the contrary, the clinical importance of this cluster division is emphasized by the result that this intermediate group presents with a significant amount of internalizing as well as externalizing, behaviorally oriented, self-harming tendencies. These patients describe significantly more self-depreciative thoughts (SNAP self-harm subscale “low self-esteem”; examples "I've really made a mess of my life", "I've wasted a lot of my life") as well as behaviors (SNAP self-harm subscale "Suicide Proneness"; examples "I sometimes wonder if I would be better off dead"; "I have hurt myself on purpose several times"). This means that these higher level BPO patients not only tend to think more about and show self-harming behaviors and suicide than the NPO patients, but also describe themselves significantly more discontent with their lives and themselves. Also, the SNAP “Impulsivity” scale, a scale expected to closely relate to self-harming behaviors, showed that the intermediate group was neither significantly different from the BPO nor from the NPO group, implying a broad range of impulsive behaviors within this cluster.

How does this finding relate to structural deficits and identity pathology in this group? In the self-reports this group did not differ significantly from the neurotic group with regard to structural deficits (e.g. on the IPO Scale “Identity diffusion” or “Primitive Defenses”), and looked significantly less disturbed than the BPO group on these scales. In other words, in this group overt pathological behaviors seem to be picked up more easily than structural deficits by the self reports. An interpretation for this discrepancy is that overt behaviors are better captured by self-reports (i.e. in this case the self-harming behaviors assessed

with the SNAP) than intrapsychic aspects (i.e. identity diffusion as assessed with the IPO).
This is one of the most important findings of this study: structural deficits seem to be captured better by an interview measure. Based on the IPO, this intermediate group did not report a high degree of identity diffusion, but different results were found based on the interview measure STIPO: almost two thirds of this intermediate group were rated with some pathology in the domain "representation of others", which is an important marker of identity diffusion. This emphasizes the need to assess these subtle intrapsychic aspects in particular by interview measures.

The discrepant findings between self-report and interview measures lead to the conclusion that these patients might be "deceptive" in a certain way: they seem healthier intrapsychically at first glance but show a significant amount of self-harming thoughts and behaviors. Translating this thought to the course of treatment one could hypothesize that these patients first seem neurotic but then, for example with the beginning of intense treatment, the behaviors turn more pathological, shown in impulsivity or self-destructive thoughts and behaviors.

The clinical implications of this result are very relevant. An early and thorough diagnosis, preferably through a clinical interview, can prevent unexpected turns once psychotherapy commences: if these patients are misdiagnosed as neurotic, they might start to become self-destructive, act out or drop out of treatment in unexpected ways. Thus, it is very beneficial to make a thorough diagnosis in advance.

When examining this intermediate group, one finding from the SNAP personality disorder scores is of particular interest. In most of the personality disorders, as measured by SNAP personality disorder symptom counts, the first cluster was significantly more disturbed than the second and third cluster. Interestingly, in narcissistic personality disorder, the second group was not significantly less disturbed than the first. This suggests that this intermediate group demonstrates a notable amount of narcissistic pathology, moving it closer to the BPO group. This is an important finding: one can postulate an association between the before-mentioned "deceptiveness" of this intermediate group with prominent narcissistic features.

This intermediate group needs to be explored further as it is interesting that these patients seem structurally less disturbed (at least when assessed by self-reports), but behaviorally show pathology that was not expected (given the fact that they described themselves in self reports closer to identity consolidation). A first conclusion is that the BPO prototype could be used to predict self-destructive behaviors in a mixed population of higher level borderline and neurotics. Furthermore, this emphasizes the need to assess structural deficits by interview measures in order to derive important treatment implications in advance.

The neurotic group

This group of patients presented to be significantly different from the first, BPO cluster on most of the measures assessing general functioning, and axis I and II pathology. This subgroup seemed similar to the intermediate group with the mentioned exception of the SNAP self-harming scale. These patients can be seen as a rather high functioning neurotic group.

1.2. Self-harm

As described in the previous section, the SNAP self-harm scale provided a meaningful differentiation between the clusters, amplifying the need to regard the second cluster as an independent group from the third. In Kernberg's model, self-harming behavior is a behavioral manifestation of underlying identity pathology. Thus, the self-harming behavior as assessed by the SNAP scale seems to be an important and sensitive indicator of borderline pathology, as found in previous research results. For example, Morey and colleagues (2003) found that the SNAP self-harm scale appeared to reflect a core trait of borderline personality disorder. In that study, mean scores for the borderline patients were quite high on this scale in comparison to any contrast group – normal, depressed, or other participants with personality disorders.

This scale seems to assess aspects of self-harming thoughts and behaviors important to BPO, that are not captured by the simple accumulation of data about a history of self-injury or suicide attempts. This data, taken from the patient charts, was analyzed in a quantitative analysis and revealed a pattern similar to the other scales: most patients with histories of self-injury were found in cluster 1, fewer in cluster 2 and none in cluster 3. Nevertheless, in the intermediate cluster, several patients reported suicide attempts in the past, which resulted in the finding of no statistically significant difference between the BPO group and the intermediate group. Also in the STIPO domain "self-directed aggression", no significant difference between the first and second cluster could be shown. This means that the intermediate and BPO cluster seem to have more pathology in common in these domains. When inspecting the intermediate cluster as it compares to the neurotic, neither the data about histories of self-injury or suicide nor the results in self-directed aggression of the STIPO did yield a significant difference between the intermediate and the neurotic cluster, differing from the results in the SNAP self-harm scale.

A possible interpretation of these findings is that self-harming thoughts and behaviors, reflecting underlying identity disturbance, are part of the core pathology that moves higher level BPO patients away from neurotic and closer to BPO patients. These variables, especially the aspect of internalizing, self-depreciating thoughts and behaviors, seem to be the most sensitive markers between the groups. In sum, these results indicate the need to explore these domains carefully to assess subtle differences in internalizing aggression, that is self-depreciating thoughts, self-injuries and suicide attempts within a mixed population of patients.

1.3. BPO prototype, subdomain "representation of others"

When inspecting the four prototypical domains across the clusters and analyzing which of the domains were scored most severely, it was shown that clearly in the subdomain "representation of others" the highest amount of patients showed deficits. Almost all of the patients in the BPO cluster, nearly two thirds in the intermediate and even one out of seven of the neurotic patients were in the prototypical range of pathology in this area (cf. figure 7). This indicates that this subdomain of identity is very sensitive in picking up pathology, not only with severely disturbed borderline patients and narcissistic patients (e.g. Kernberg, 1984) but also with neurotic patients.

It should be noted that for the two domains "object relations" and "primitive defenses" a higher cut-off for prototypicality was chosen. This might explain

why fewer patients were in the prototypical realm in these domains. But especially in relation to the other subdomain of Identity, "coherence of self" (which had the same cut-off as "representation of others"), "representation of others" seemed to be more sensitive in capturing pathology. Many of the patients had great difficulties describing others so the interviewers could obtain a full picture of the object; also the patients said they had problems assessing others or had an unclear view about what others thought about them.
The range of pathology in this STIPO domain was demonstrated by the four single cases illustrated in the second part of the results, in which the patient with strong antisocial traits demonstrated severe pathology (score of 5), both the borderline patient and the patient with narcissistic traits showed moderate pathology (score of 3) and the neurotic patient absence of pathology (score of 1).

The finding that representation of others seems more sensitive than representation of self in picking up pathology of identity and internal object relations is very important for the diagnosis of personality pathology: difficulties in the perception and understanding of others could become a key domain when diagnosing identity and hence for the diagnosis and differential diagnosis of various levels of personality pathology. This result should be examined with a larger sample of patients at various levels of pathology.

1.4. <u>Interrater reliability of the BPO prototype (Hypothesis 2)</u>

Interrater reliability for the four clinical ratings of the BPO prototype, based on a subgroup of the clinical sample, was very high. This is an important finding when taking into consideration that this study is examining the ratings based on the clinical impression of the raters, as opposed to the item-level ratings which were examined elsewhere (Stern et al., 2007). The high interrater reliability could be explained by the small sample size and the extensive training the raters went through, and needs to be replicated in future studies with larger samples. In sum, finding high interrater reliability on the clinical scales of the STIPO is an encouraging finding given the fact that this instrument operationalizes a psychodynamic theory.

1.5. Validity of the BPO similarity index (Hypotheses 3-5)

When examining the convergent and incremental validity of the BPO similarity index, encouraging results were found through different statistical analyses.

Convergent validity

Regarding convergent validity, as hypothesized, the BPO similarity index correlated highly with measures of axis II like the SNAP diagnostic scales and with correlates of axis II like SNAP temperament scales, measures of aggression and hostility and with measures of negative affectivity. Also, an inverse correlation between the index and measures not expected to be part of BPO was found, for example measures of positive affect or agreeableness. This is in line with the results which show that borderline pathology is characterized by a prominence of negative versus positive affect and that borderline patients have difficulties in experiencing pleasure (Kernberg, 1984; Lenzenweger et al., 2001).

Part of the examination of the convergent validity was the association with the individual DSM personality disorders. The BPO similarity index correlated comparably high with the dimensional scores of the SNAP diagnostic scales from all of the different DSM clusters, for example with paranoid personality disorder, BPD and dependent personality disorder. This indicates that the conceptualization of a prototype of the broad spectrum Borderline Personality Organization that cuts across the individual DSM personality disorders and clusters was confirmed. An interesting finding is that the BPO similarity index and the diagnostic scale of BPD correlate highly. Also the aforementioned result is notable: that the BPO index and the self-harm scale correlate highest of all measures of axis II pathology (besides the association between BPD and self-harm). Together this might imply that the broadly conceptualized BPO concept is very close to BPD and to one of the core traits of BPD, that is self-harm (Morey et al., 2003; Shearer, 1994; Soloff et al., 1994).

Aggression

In Kernberg's model of BPO, aggression plays a crucial role in the development of both identity diffusion and primitive defenses (1984; Kernberg, 1975; 1996). The association of aggression with the BPO index was confirmed. First, the index showed a very high correlation with the SNAP subscale “Self-harm”, which indicates a strong link between the BPO prototype and self-directed aggression. Also, with measures assessing other-directed aggression, for example the PANAS “Hostility” scale and the IPO “Aggression” scale, as well as the Buss-Durkee “Irritability” scale, the index could account for additional variance after variance accounted for by the BFI and IPO was removed. This does indicate an association between the STIPO prototype and these measures of hostility. On the other hand, no additional variance in the SNAP subscale “Aggression” could be accounted for by the index after the variance explained through 1) the BFI and 2) the IPO was partialed out. A possible explanation for these findings could be that the index did not include the STIPO domain “Aggression”, therefore a lower association might be expected and was found with the SNAP domain “Aggression”. In contrast, the prototype did pick up on hostile and aggressive traits and correlates when examined in relation to other measures of aggression and hostility. The Buss-Durkee scale is conceptualized to assess aggressive dyscontrol, which according to Lenzenweger et al. (2001) probably also involves some element of negative affect (which itself correlated highly with the BPO index). Thus, the correlation of the index with irritability as conceptualized by the Buss Durkee scale corresponds to the remaining findings; and aggression as assessed by the SNAP, might be of different content.

Incremental validity

When examining the incremental validity of the BPO index, it could be shown that the index was able to explain additional portions of variance in symptoms and correlates of BPO after the variance explained by a measure of the Five-Factor-Model of Personality (FFM) was partialed out. The interpretation of these results, for example, with regard to the SNAP BPD scale, SNAP self-harm scale or the IPO aggression scale is that the BPO index seemed to capture important elements of borderline pathology which the FFM did not. Again, the closeness of the BPO prototype to the BPD concept and to aggression is striking and confirms, at least regarding these variables, the strength of the theory-based model over an atheoretical model like the FFM.

Finally, another aspect of incremental validity of the BPO index was investigated. The BPO index could explain moderate amounts of additional variance in axis II symptoms (e.g. SNAP BPD scale, SNAP avoidant personality disorder scale) and correlates (e.g. PANAS Negative Affect Scale) after variance explained through the self-report IPO was partialed out. This is an important finding regarding the validation of the STIPO. As the IPO is the self-report precursor of the interview STIPO and is based on the same theoretical conceptions, a high overlap is expected and was confirmed in this study: This demonstrates construct validity for the domains of BPO as conceptualized by Kernberg.

Furthermore, it is of great interest to find additional variance explained by the interview measure (i.e. BPO similarity index based on the STIPO) over the self-report. These results are encouraging, especially when considering that all the self-report measures (e.g. SNAP, IPO, IIP-PD) share method variance. Given that the outcome measures of this analysis and the STIPO do not share method variance, one might expect the predictive power to be less. The fact that incremental validity was still found can be seen as a very important result for the validation of the BPO prototype and of the STIPO.

As the BPO prototype, consisting of two subscales of the identity domain, the object relations domain and the primitive defenses domain, can be considered to be a short version of the STIPO, these results are encouraging for the further development of the STIPO.

2 Integration

2.1. Implications for the diagnosis of personality pathology

Prototypical domains

For the classification of personality pathology, one of the key domains that Kernberg builds on is identity diffusion. Identity is the cornerstone of his model of personality organization. It is the degree of identity disturbance that distinguishes patients with severe personality disorders from neurotic patients. The findings in this study confirm the relevance of assessing identity and identity disturbance. The BPO-prototypical domains consisting of aspects of identity diffusion, as well as disturbed object relations and predominance of primitive defenses, were found to be important and differentially valuable in the diagnosis of borderline personality pathology.

It is interesting to note that two important aspects of identity diffusion assessed with the STIPO were proven valuable for diagnosis. These are difficulties in the *sense of self*, but also difficulties in the *representation of others*. Kernberg emphasizes not only the absence of a stable sense of self, but also the lack of internalized object representations, to be crucial elements of identity diffusion (Kernberg, 1976). These unintegrated object representations are assessed in the STIPO domain "representation of others". The strong sensitivity of this domain in picking up pathology, perhaps even more so than "sense of self" is a quite relevant finding. The importance of the individual's representation of others is well in line with the findings of Fonagy and his group regarding the significance of mentalization, i.e. the capacity to envision mental states in self and others, for pathological self-development and personality pathology (Bateman & Fonagy, 2004b; Fonagy & Target, 1997; Fonagy, Target & Gergely, 2000).

Thus, assessing difficulties in the perception of self and others, as well as the predominance of primitive defenses and disturbed object relations, including friendships and intimate relationships, were shown to be differentially important for the structure-oriented diagnostic process. The assessment of these areas is assumed to capture similar elements as the structural diagnosis done by the KAPP (Weinryb & Rossel, 1991), the OPD axis "structure" (Arbeitskreis OPD, 1996; 2006; OPD Task Force, 2001) or the Scales of Psychological Capacities (Huber, Klug & Wallerstein, 2006; Wallerstein, 1991) which would be an interesting area for future research.

Structural diagnosis

One of the research questions of this study was to investigate how much a dimensional assessment of variables central to Kernberg's model of personality pathology – with an emphasis on the structural criteria of identity and internal object relations – can complement or add to a categorical diagnosis focusing primarily on symptoms. Focusing on structural deficits or levels of personality organization has been reported as being helpful in the diagnostic process (e.g. Kernberg, 1984; Lohmer, 1988). Then, some authors have criticized that there is a risk of clinicians diagnosing structural deficits too rashly, and moving from a thorough psychoanalytically oriented process to a mainly descriptive one. For example, Weidenhammer (1987, cit. in Mertens, 1992) points out that the process of decision making and diagnosing is susceptible to rash decisions when

interviewing patients with structural deficits; and that, instead of solely stating deficiencies, it is of high importance to explore the transference-countertransference interaction and to conduct an extensive psychodynamic interview.
This is an important aspect of the diagnostic process according to Kernberg, especially in the Structural Interview, where the interviewer is urged to follow elements of perceived transference-countertransference processes and to integrate these in the diagnostic method, and to not only focus on symptoms. The STIPO, aiming at higher reliability between different raters, provides less flexibility or freedom to follow these transference- countertransference leads (than for example the Structural Interview), as it has a clear structure and order of questions. Notably, the STIPO does allow the interviewer to weigh in his clinical impression to a certain degree, by confronting inconsistencies when it appears that the answer contradicts other data or appears to be superficial.
This means that the STIPO provides a rather structured approach which still enables the interviewer to incorporate his clinical impression to a certain degree, especially in the clinical 5-point ratings. The goal of developing the instrument and BPO prototype was to make it possible for interviewers less familiar with the theoretical background and less experienced in interviewing to establish a reliable structural diagnosis.

In this study, the thorough investigation and focus on aspects relevant to the assessment of structure (i.e., the prototypical domains) has proven valuable for the diagnosis of patients. When examining the results from the present sample by looking at the number of diagnoses by the categorical scoring method in the SNAP (which is in line with the DSM diagnostic process), it can be seen that the frequencies of SNAP categorical diagnoses of lower level personality disorders (DSM cluster A or B) were rather low in the BPO cluster (less than half of the patients fulfilled the criteria for one of these diagnoses). In contrast, this cluster was highly pathological in structural aspects like identity diffusion or use of primitive defenses as assessed by the IPO, and, of course, as shown by the fulfilled BPO prototypical dimensions. The structural diagnosis derived from the BPO prototype seemed meaningful, due to its ability to differentiate between clinical groups and also due to its high correlation with important BPO correlates like negative affect. This means that the assessment of structural deficits by the BPO prototype seems to be more "sensitive" than the personality disorder diagnoses alone. A consequential thought could be to combine an interview focusing on psychological structure (e.g. the STIPO) with a symptom-oriented instrument (e.g. SCID-II; First et al., 1996)in order to obtain a thorough assessment and diagnosis of the patient.

Interview measure versus self-report

In a study on the extent to which instruments assessing axis II pathology diverge from clinical diagnostic processes, Westen (1997) concluded that personality pathology is difficult to assess with instruments like structured interviews and questionnaires. As measurements of axis II were constructed by using a model derived from axis I instruments, these assessments were primarily based on questions about axis II criteria and presumed that patients had insight and the ability to report on their internal processes. He reported that practicing clinicians therefore often preferred to assess personality pathology by listening to the narratives patients told about their lives or observing the behaviors the patients exhibited during the interview.

This again elicits the need to incorporate clinical judgment in the diagnostic process of axis II pathology and shows how important it is for the clinician to pose additional questions during the assessment procedure to deepen his understanding of what the patient reports. Also, in an interview the diagnostician has the opportunity to explore further when he believes the patient does not reply honestly. According to Blatt, honest replies depend on several aspects; the patient's willingness to share and engage with the therapist, the patient's degree of reflectiveness and the social desirability of the behavior under question (S. Blatt, personal communication, April 22, 2004). These factors have a strong influence on the way the patient will frame his responses, which cannot be explored further when given in a self-report format, but can be tested thoroughly in an interview. For example, in an interview like the Structural Interview or the STIPO, the interviewer is asked to confront the patient if he clearly sounds inconsistent (e.g. due to social desirable response patterns), thus providing the interviewer with a certain flexibility in the diagnostic process.

In this study, we can compare the results based on an interview designed to assess axis II pathology with the results from several self-report measures. It is interesting to note that based on the STIPO, more patients were diagnosed as BPO- prototypical, i.e. presenting personality pathology in the STIPO domains than when compared to the results from the self report SNAP diagnostic scales. Indicating that the BPO prototype, assessed through the STIPO, is more sensitive in picking up pathology in the interpersonal domain than the self-report, this suggests the added usefulness of an interview measure, designed to detect interpersonal pathology, over a self-report measure. This finding is especially encouraging when taking into consideration the high interrater reliability found for the interview, in particular when considering that the STIPO builds on a psychodynamic theory.

Obviously, a questionnaire is very time efficient, and it might be considered the goal of profound assessment to combine both approaches to complement each other in order to achieve a valid diagnosis of the personality pathology. For example, Zimmerman and colleagues propose using both an interview measure as well as a self administered questionnaire, which can serve as a paper standard with which interviewer-derived diagnoses can be compared (Zimmerman, 1994; Zimmerman, Coryell & Black, 1993).

For the development and validation of the STIPO, the concurrent use of the interview STIPO and the self-report IPO has shown to be very valuable, in particular by demonstrating incremental validity of the STIPO-based BPO similarity index over the IPO. Also, it is important that future research will further examine the construct validity of Kernberg's concepts, which was indicated in this study by similar findings across the different assessment methods. The finding of a close fit between both instruments and the theory they operationalize is one of the key findings of this study.

Differential diagnosis

One of the primary goals of this study was to develop a prototype of BPO which could differentiate between *borderline* and *neurotic* personality. The results indicate that the BPO prototype is also able to differentiate between *different levels of borderline* personality organization. The level of identity diffusion versus identity consolidation, captured by each patient's similarity to the BPO prototype, is an important differential marker for diagnosis and treatment. The intermediate cluster, consisting of higher level BPO patients, was separated from the majority of lower level BPO patients in the first cluster.

In the BPO cluster, many patients were diagnosed with several co-occurring SNAP personality disorders. This corresponds to the finding of high co-occurrence of personality disorders (e.g. Oldham et al., 1992; Zimmerman, Rothschild, & Chelminski, 2005). Often, the usefulness of these multiple diagnoses is questioned. Especially when aiming at differential diagnosis in order to derive treatment implications, it might be more helpful to look at the overall level of personality pathology and the structural level, as well as specific deficits and ressources, not at the individual diagnoses. Hence, in addition to the symptom-oriented categorical diagnoses, the BPO prototype can guide important treatment planning thoughts.

These implications were exemplified by the four individual patients described in the single case section. They represent different levels of pathology in the STIPO, which was assessed through their similarity to the prototype. The first patient showed severe pathology in the sense of self, moderate pathology in the representation of others, as well as severe problems in her object relations and defense mechanisms, and was located on a lower level of personality organization (Borderline 2). As she presented a certain concern about her situation and showed no severe antisocial traits, a psychoanalytic psychotherapy like TFP was recommended for her. The second patient demonstrated very severe pathology in most of the prototypical domains, plus severe other directed aggression and absence of internalized moral values, and was located at the lowest level of personality organization (Borderline 3 in the STIPO). She was given a poor prognosis and the perspective for this patient to benefit from psychotherapy was very limited. The third patient (Borderline 1) was a higher level borderline patient with narcissistic features, who fulfilled only two of the four prototypic criteria, namely identity difficulties (i.e. impairment both with sense of self and sense of others), but was supported by important object relations, and who presented a mixed pattern of using primitive defenses. Although slightly limited capacity for insight was stated, he showed some motivation to change and psychoanalytic psychotherapy (e.g. TFP) was recommended. The fourth patient was located at neurotic personality organization (Neurotic 1 in the STIPO). Her problems differed from the other three patients (namely in the area of self-worth, depression and a self demanding, slightly overambitious personality style), and she did not show a significant amount of pathology in any of the BPO prototypical dimensions. In her case, a treatment for neurotic personality came into question, for example psychoanalysis. Hence, these examples show how the BPO prototype can help in the differential diagnosis and treatment choice.

An interesting finding regarding the individual patients is that the narcissistic patient (patient 3) is part of the first cluster (albeit in one of the healthier subgroups of this cluster) which is characterized by disturbance of identity, object relations and use of primitive defenses. The finding that this patient is part of the BPO cluster supports Kernberg's concept of narcissistic pathology: lower level narcissistic patients can present as comparably disturbed as patients with Borderline Personality Disorder and can be diagnosed through clinical-descriptive criteria. This finding contrasts with Kohut's self-psychological model (1971) of narcissistic patients not being as severely disturbed and primarily being differentiated from others through their transference manifestations.

2.2. <u>Implications for treatment choice, prognosis and therapy</u>

The question of differential indication for treatments, for example deciding on a patient's suitability for psychoanalysis versus psychoanalytic psychotherapy versus other therapy forms, has been discussed intensely throughout the years. Mertens (1992) mentions several questions which play a role in deciding on the appropriate treatment: are some disorders especially suitable for psychoanalysis, or do specific disorders exclude the choice of psychoanalytic treatment? In addition to the disorder, do specific traits or motivations play an important role, or is the "analyzability" or ability to "mentalize" one of the key aspects? How can the suitability and analyzability reliably be judged in the first psychoanalytic interview? Also, does the role of the diagnostician and his reactions have a strong influence on diagnosis and treatment choice? The purpose of finding a treatment which corresponds to the patient's needs and abilities leads to the goal of an adaptive process which still takes into account the classical indications for treatment.

In Kernberg's theory, the degree of identity consolidation determines the level of personality organization. Treatment choice, as well as prognosis clearly depend on it. For example, psychoanalysis is recommended only if the patient's ego is strong enough to sustain the decomposition of the personality into its component object relations units and subsequent reintegration of them into a new structure. This is not the case for BPO, but for neurotic personality organization. For patients located at BPO, Kernberg recommends psychodynamic psychotherapy like TFP (Clarkin, Yeomans, & Kernberg, 2006).

For a thorough decision on the appropriate treatment, the assessment of the level of personality organization is necessary, as done by the STIPO and the BPO prototype. One of the key findings stemming from this study is the ability of the STIPO and BPO prototype to aid in the choice of the appropriate treatment and to provide information which can help to establish a prognosis. As mentioned in the previous section and described at length in the single case section, the individual's similarity to the BPO prototype aids in diagnosing patients according to their structural deficits and is of assistance in the treatment decision process and development of foci for psychotherapy. For example, focusing on self and object representations during the assessment gives important hints when deciding on the ability to "mentalize" or the "analyzability" of the patient. Strong impairment in analyzability, as shown in most patients with structural deficits, indicate that these patients are not suitable for psychoanalysis in its classical form, but that insight-oriented, modified psychotherapeutic treatments like TFP might be more appropriate.

From the single cases, the neurotic patient was clearly considered able to undergo insight-oriented psychotherapy or psychoanalysis. For the individual patients located at Borderline level 1 and 2, insight-oriented treatments were considered, whilst the patient at Borderline level 1 was considered to be in more stable relationships which might be a good prognostic factor. The severely disturbed second patient (Borderline level 3) demonstrated lack of insight, complete disinterest in others, paired with aggression, secondary gain and antisocial traits and thus was not regarded as suitable for that kind of therapy.

When establishing the prognosis for a patient and the expectations from the therapy process, several aspects are important according to Kernberg's theory.

In particular, the degree of super-ego integration is an enormously important structural criterion for the indication or counterindication of long-term, intensive psychotherapy. Kernberg (1984) states that the quality of object relations and the quality of super-ego functioning are probably the two most important prognostic criteria stemming from a structural analysis. Thus, in the diagnostic situation, besides secondary gain and motivation for treatment, the quality of object relations, the intensity of aggression and maturity of the superego are crucial prognostic criteria which the diagnostician should focus on (Kernberg & Caligor, 2005). Regarding the diagnosis of superego integration and aggression, interesting results were found in a larger sample of BPO patients (Stern et al., 2007). It could be shown that the STIPO sections "moral values" and "aggression" (which were not part of the BPO prototype in this study) were useful in discriminating among the healthier and more severely personality disordered patients within a larger sample of BPO patients. These criteria, along with other results from the diagnostic process, will help inform the clinician's decision regarding treatment choice. Future research could follow up on the subgroups according to the aspects considered prognostically relevant and examine each subgroup's treatment process and outcome.

The results from the STIPO during the diagnostic phase can provide a decision tree for foci in the subsequent psychodynamic treatment. Once the four prototypical domains are assessed, it is likely to become clear where one must probe for further evaluation. Also, in these four domains we expect the clinician to have derived important elements which can guide the treatment. For example, the assessment of the domain "representation of others" will help to determine what kind of difficulties the patient has in understanding and interacting with others. This can also facilitate assessing the therapeutic relationship and deducing the possible course of treatment.

2.3. <u>Development of the STIPO</u>

The development and validation of the STIPO is still in process. Preliminary results indicate that the STIPO is an instrument with good internal consistency and interrater reliability which can be used to determine different levels of pathology within a clinical sample (Stern et al., 2004a; 2004b;2007).

An aspect taken into consideration for the further development of the STIPO is the use of the two rating systems employed in the present version of the interview. As exemplified in the single case section of this study, for the most part, the overlap between the STIPO 0-2 ratings with the 1-5 ratings was rather high. Also, it was shown that the similarity indices based on the two ratings systems correlated highly with each other, indicating a strong association between the 0-2 ratings and the 1-5 ratings. The two different rating systems will be examined in the further development of the instrument.

The reliability and validity of the BPO prototype, based on the clinical ratings of the STIPO, has been confirmed. It has been shown that four domains, which are part of the overall STIPO, can be used to assess different levels of personality organization; discriminating between BPO and NPO, but also between different levels of BPO. As this is one of the goals of the STIPO, the development and validation of the BPO prototype – which can essentially be regarded a "short version" of the STIPO – has been an important step in the development and validation of the STIPO as a whole.

A practical implication could be to use the four prototypical domains as a "screening version" of the STIPO. These domains, the sense of self and others, the nature and quality of object relations and the use of primitive defensive operations, operationalize Kernberg's main components of borderline personality organization. One could use these STIPO questions as the first step in a diagnostic process. If these four domains indicate at which level of personality organization the patient is located, the choice and foci of treatment can be guided by these results. Then, further exploration based on the remaining STIPO domains, for example "Moral Values" and "Aggression", can be considered. For example, the remaining STIPO domains can be carried out in a subsequent interview session in order to yield a detailed personality profile. Overall, the "short version" based on the prototype domains could be used as a condensed interview.

3 Limitations, conclusions and future

Interview measures

One of the basic limitations of this study is the fact that no personality disorders interview was included. Because of time considerations and to avoid overburdening the patients, only one interview, the rather extensive STIPO, was conducted and the other measures were assessed in self-report format. Another interview measure of personality disorders would be helpful in comparing the interview-based diagnosis of DSM personality disorders with STIPO-based assessment of personality pathology. For the present study, sufficient information on personality disorders was expected from the results of the SNAP diagnostic scales. Clark (1993) reports that the SNAP personality disorders scales are highly correlated with the "Structured Interview for DSM-III-R Personality" (SIDP-R) (Pfohl et al., 1989).
The findings of the cross-method convergence in this study are encouraging, in particular between the interview-based BPO prototype and the self-report-based assessment of personality pathology, but need to be confirmed further. Replicating this study using standardized interview measures like the SCID-II (First et al., 1996) would be very useful when inspecting the STIPO's validity in explaining variance in personality pathology. This would be particularly interesting for the examination of the mutual relationships of the DSM personality disorders and Kernberg's higher-level and lower level personality disorders as assessed by the BPO prototype. Future studies should investigate the association of structural aspects as assessed by the STIPO and interview based diagnosis of personality disorders based on the DSM categorization.

Another limitation is that due to time constraints, the dimensions of the Five-Factor-Model of Personality were assessed by the rather short self-report BFI-44. It is not as detailed as the NEO-PI-R or NEO-FFI (Costa & McCrae, 1992b), but correlates highly with these instruments (John, Donahue, & Kentle, 1991).

Sample size

Generalizations based on the results of this study have to be done carefully due to the small sample size (N=60), in particular of the subgroup of less disturbed patients (n= 10) and patients clearly falling into the neurotic spectrum of personality organization (n=7). Future studies need to comprise large sample sizes, especially more heterogenic clinical groups including higher-functioning patients, to test the ability of the prototype and of the STIPO to portray the whole spectrum of personality functioning. Examining the performance of the STIPO with a sample of high functioning patients (as was done for example by Westen & Shedler, 1999a) would provide important insights as to the differential validity of the instrument. It is encouraging to note that in the first validation study of the IPO by Lenzenweger and colleagues (2001), which is the self-report precursor of the STIPO, a large non-clinical sample was examined and the results correspond in many respects to the results from this study.

Future research

Future research could use the STIPO and an external measure of Axis II pathology in a larger sample in order to test the cut-offs in the four STIPO-based prototypical domains. As the cut-offs in this study were theory-based they could be examined in a larger sample of pre-formed groups of different levels of personality pathology. The goal would be to establish optimal cut-off scores for clinical groups in the BPO prototype by this method. This way the ability of the BPO prototype and the STIPO of distinguishing between BPO, NPO and normal personality organization would be studied further.

An interesting field of future research is the association of the BPO prototype and the STIPO with other instruments aiming at the assessment of psychic structure and structural change. Studies using several interviews could provide meaningful results for the construct validity of the STIPO. For example, analyzing the association of the BPO prototype and "structure" as assessed by the OPD (Arbeitskreis OPD, 2006; Grande et al., 2001; Rudolf, Oberbracht, & Grande, 1998) might be particularly useful in validating the assessment of different structural levels, as is the goal of the STIPO based prototype. Another interesting focus of future research could be the association between structural level as assessed by the STIPO and the degree of mentalization, which is conceptualized as the ability to make sense of each other and oneself, implicitly and explicitly in terms of subjective states and mental processes (Bateman & Fonagy, 2004a). The degree of mentalization, operationalized by the "Reflective Functioning Scale" by Fonagy and colleagues (1998) and the structural level assessed by the STIPO could be assessed in patients with and without personality disorders, in order to examine the overlap between these two measures. Coming from two different theoretical and research backgrounds, the level of correspondence is expected to be very interesting. Likewise, the association between degree of identity pathology, measured by the STIPO and the attachment classification, assessed for example by the AAI (George, Kaplan & Main, 1985) could be another noteworthy research question. Bringing together information regarding personality pathology and attachment style could provide important implications for the course and outcome of psychotherapy, as has been discussed for the measures separately (e.g. Dahlbender, Buchheim & Doering, 2004; Fonagy et al., 1996).

Yet another research question would be to study the association between the STIPO and the "Scales of Psychological Capacities" (Huber, Klug, & Wallerstein, 2006; Wallerstein, 1991), in particular when examining the question of structural change. Both instruments could be applied before and after psychotherapy and their convergence and assessment of structural change could be compared.

Clinical conclusions

Addressing the clinician's work, some important conclusions can be drawn from this study. The confirmation of a prototype of BPO and the finding that most BPO patients share specific deficits, can help clinicians focus on the most relevant aspects of BPO when diagnosing patients. Carrying out only the four prototypical domains of the interview (i.e. a shorter version of the STIPO) can be of high interest for the clinician's day to day work; especially when considering the duration of the complete interview. The BPO prototypical dimensions could serve as diagnostic templates against which an individual's profile is compared to assess degree of match, i.e. the closeness to the prototype in the four prototypical domains, using the five-point scale from (1) to (5). Then, the threshold for the categorical assignment of the diagnosis "BPO" versus "NPO" would depend upon the cutoffs of the prototypical domain scores. This way, both a dimensional (closeness to prototype) and categorical assessment (above-threshold vs. below-threshold in the domains) could be made. Once the level of pathology in these areas is identified, and the patient's similarity to the prototype assessed, this information could be utilized for differential treatment planning and to help target specific areas for treatment.

The construct of identity as the cornerstone of Kernberg's theory and the STIPO was examined in this study. Four domains from the STIPO, attempting to operationalize the concept of identity, were inspected as to their utility in the diagnosis of personality pathology. The usefulness of this approach was confirmed. This could be regarded a pilot study and should be replicated with a large sample and several instruments, combining self-report and interview measures. The further validation of the STIPO will be an important step for the diagnostic assessment of personality pathology and the option of using the BPO prototype as a short version or screening version of this instrument will be considered.

VII SUMMARY

The diagnosis of personality pathology based on Kernberg's psychoanalytic theory of personality organization (Kernberg, 1975; 1976; 1984) was examined in this study. Kernberg's model classifies personality according to levels of psychic structure, focusing on the construct of identity. The Structured Interview of Personality Organization (Clarkin et al., 2004) was developed as an outgrowth of Kernberg's "Structural Interview" and as a way of operationalizing Kernberg's theory. In this study, domains from the STIPO were used to generate a prototype of Borderline Personality Organization (BPO), and its utility in explaining variance in personality pathology across a sample of patients of different levels of pathology was examined.

Experts on Kernberg's theory formed a consensus about which of the STIPO domains should be included in a BPO prototype that would differentiate between Borderline Personality Organization (BPO) and Neurotic Personality Organization (NPO). Using these STIPO domains, a prototypical profile of BPO was created and tested for clinical usefulness and psychometric properties.

The results of this study show that four prototypical areas of BPO could be identified in which all borderline personality patients present similar difficulties. The prototypic BPO profile consisted of STIPO domains assessing pathology in "Identity – sense of self", "Identity – sense of others", "Object Relations", and "Primitive Defenses". This BPO prototype was able to discriminate between clinically relevant groups according to levels of pathology in general functioning, axis I and II symptoms and correlates. By means of a hierarchical cluster analysis, a BPO group, a NPO group and a meaningful intermediate group were found. Differences between the groups in general functioning and variables of axis I and II pathology (assessed by a set of self report measures, e.g. BSI, SNAP, PANAS) were examined by one-way analyses of variance.

High interrater reliability was obtained for the clinical ratings of the four prototypical STIPO domains. Also, the BPO prototype was examined with regard to its validity. By matching the similarity of 60 patients of a clinical sample to the BPO prototype, a BPO similarity index was computed. It correlated highly with measures of axis II symptoms and correlates (e.g. SNAP borderline personality disorder scale; PANAS negative affect Scale, SNAP self-harm scale), thus establishing its convergent validity.

The incremental validity of the BPO similarity index was confirmed in a hierarchical regression analysis by explaining additional variance in measures of axis I and II pathology over a measure of the Five-Factor-Model of personality. This finding emphasizes the usefulness of a theory-derived assessment of personality pathology. The ability of the BPO similarity index to explain additional variance over the Inventory of Personality Organization (Clarkin, Foelsch, & Kernberg, 2001), the self-report precursor of the STIPO, further established its incremental validity. This result indicates the usefulness of the interview measure in addition to the self report measure. This also demonstrates cross-method construct validity of the assessed content, i.e. the domains of the instruments aiming at identity pathology, commensurate with Kernberg's theory.

Four individual cases of different degrees of pathology and similarity to the BPO prototype (Borderline 1, Borderline 2, Borderline 3 and Neurotic 1 as assessed by the STIPO) were presented to exemplify the STIPO and the four prototypical domains. The STIPO personality profiles of these individuals were related to other measures of general functioning and personality pathology. Finally, the results were used to describe implications regarding prognosis and treatment.

The theory-based prototype of BPO is considered useful for the diagnosis of individual patients and in explaining personality pathology in this clinical sample. As the BPO prototype is based on domains of the Structured Interview of Personality Organization, this instrument can be regarded important for the operationalization of Kernberg's theory of personality organization, which focuses on the construct of identity. The BPO prototype and STIPO can be seen as valuable tools for the diagnosis of patients with personality pathology and for deriving corresponding treatment implications.

VIII APPENDICES

1 Tables and figures

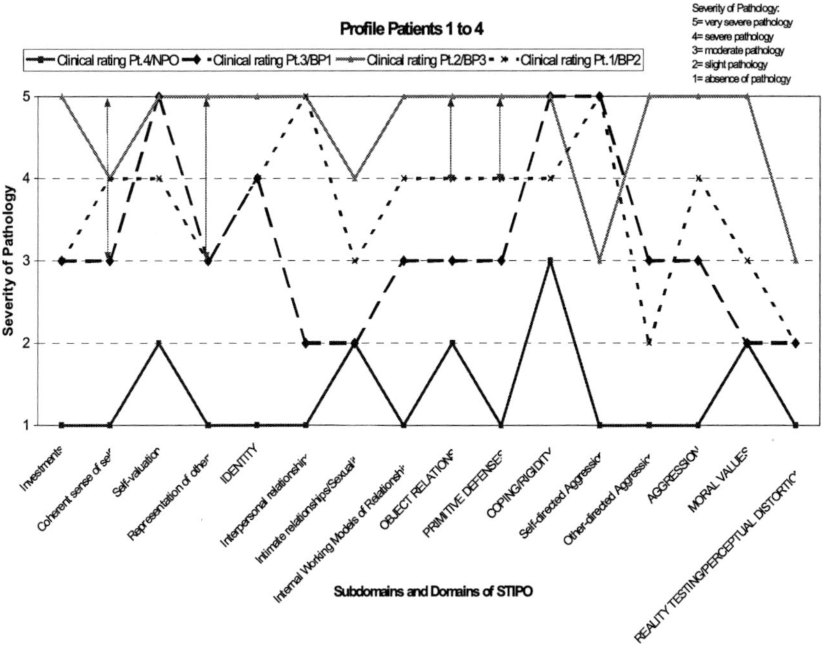

Figure 61. STIPO profiles of the four patients

4	5	6	7	8	9	10	11	12	13	14	15	16	17	18	19	20
-																
.51*	-															
.67**	.77**	-														
.49**	.72**	.65**	-													
.12	.46**	.37**	.59*	-												
.75**	.30*	.47**	.20	-.24	-											
.54**	.29*	.59**	.22	.10	.48*	-										
.44**	.34**	.47**	.46*	.29*	.42*	.21	-									
.56**	.33**	.57**	.24	-.01	.56*	.63**	.41*	-								
.54**	.44**	.56**	.36*	.03	.49*	.50**	.42*	.81*	-							
.69**	.47**	.78**	.43*	.24	.60*	.66**	.52*	.68*	.62**	-						
.60**	.65**	.73**	.61*	.37**	.38*	.38**	.37*	.39*	.53**	.64*	-					
.44**	.57**	.65**	.34*	.24	.31*	.39**	.01	.37*	.38**	.38*	.49**	-				
.65**	.48**	.82**	.40*	.11	.59*	.62**	.45*	.59*	.59**	.76*	.54**	.50*	-			
.59**	.57**	.72**	.42*	.21	.47*	.51**	.39*	.60*	.59**	.72*	.73**	.53*	.53**	-		
.67**	.59**	.75**	.64*	.33**	.45*	.44**	.37*	.49*	.52**	.63*	.79**	.48*	.64**	.64*	-	
.73**	.58**	.74**	.57*	.31**	.46*	.57**	.35*	.57*	.57**	.63*	.68**	.50*	.62**	.67*	.70**	-

	1	2	3
1.IIP-PD	-		
2.Par PD	.75*	-	
3.Schiz PD	.28*	.50**	-
4.Schizotyp PD	.73*	.87**	.64**
5.Antisoc PD	.62*	.59**	.29*
6.BPD	.75*	.70**	.33*
7.Narc PD	.60*	.52**	.22
8.Histr. PD	.28*	.13	-.24
9.Av PD	.44*	.54**	.81**
10.Dep PD	.53*	.64**	.13
11.Obs PD	.46*	.38**	.34**
12. PANAS Neg.Aff.	.57*	.58**	.32*
13. PANAS Host.	.59*	.59**	.34**
14. SNAP Neg Temp	.68*	.72**	.33**
15. SNAP Agg.	.73*	.72**	.29*
16. SNAP Impuls.	.51*	.41**	.28*
17. SNAP Self-Harm	.58*	.60**	.44*
18. Buss-D Irr.	.74*	.70**	.30*
19. IPO Agression	.74*	.70**	.33**
20. IPO Prim Def	.81*	.70**	.26*

** $p < .01$.; * $p < .05$; *Note*: Var. 2 through 11 are SNAP Personality Disorders Subscales

Table 23. Convergent Validity of the BPO Index. Correlations between measures of axis II pathology and correlates of axis II conditions (N=60)

2 STIPO Score Form

STRUCTURED INTERVIEW FOR PERSONALITY ORGANZATION (STIPO)

SCORE FORM

John F. Clarkin, Eve Caligor, Barry L. Stern & Otto F. Kernberg

Personality Disorders Institute
Weill Medical College of Cornell University

Interviewee Participant #:	________________
Interviewee Gender:	__M __ F
Interviewee Age:	________________
Interviewee Marital Status:	________________
Interviewee's Children (# of children and ages)	________________
	________________
Interviewer Name:	________________
Interview Date:	________________

IDENTITY

Investments

Work – effectiveness	1. ______
Work – stability	2. ______
Work – Ambition/goals	3. ______
Work – satisfaction	4. ______
Studies – effectiveness	5. ______
Studies – stability	6. ______
Studies – enjoyment	7. ______
Studies – correspondence	8. ______
Recreation – has interests	9. ______
Recreation – sustained interest	10. ______
Recreation – satisfaction	11. ______

Investments Overall ______

1 Invests over time and consistently in work or studies, and free time activities
2 Invests in some areas but not others; may invest in all areas but with a greater sense of superficiality and lesser commitment than in #1
3 Inconsistent, superficial investment in work/studies/free time; may have more solid investment in one area, but generally not in others
4 Minimal investment in work or studies or free time; severely deficient in two or more of these areas, even if solidly invested in one area
5 No investment in work, studies, free time

Sense of Self

Sense of self: Coherence and continuity	
Self – description	12. _____
Self - consistency across time	13. _____
Self - tastes / opinions	14. _____
Self- consistent sense of self in present	15. _____
Self- time alone	16. _____
Self – in intimate relationship	17. _____

Sense of self : Coherence and continuity ______

1 Self experience and life goals are coherent and continuous across time and situation
2 Self experience and life goals are generally coherent and continuous across time and situation
3 Self experience is superficial and unstable with an unclear sense of a self across situations and time
4 Poorly integrated and unstable experience of self
5 Unintegrated and chaotic (incoherent) self experience with no sense of having a "self"

<u>Sense of self: Self-valuation</u>

Self – self valuation	18. _____
Self – positive comparative self valuation	19. _____
Self – negative comparative self valuation	20. _____
Self – self-esteem fluctuation	21. _____
Self - self-esteem external influence	22. _____

Sense of self: Self valuation ______

1 Self -esteem is relatively stable, positive, and realistic
2 Self -esteem is stable, somewhat negative, somewhat realistic
3 Faulty self -esteem maintenance, with a tendency to experience oneself positively or negatively, largely through comparisons with others
4 Sense of self organized around needing to experience self as superior to others, alternating with feelings of self -loathing and worthlessness
5 Self -esteem is highly unrealistic, extreme, polarized, rigid views of self, positive or negative ,based on inner need to see oneself as either better or worse than others; almost a psychotic quality to these perceptions in that they are impervious to reality testing

<u>Representation of Others</u>

Other – description	23. _____
Other – assessing others	24. _____
Other – other's judgments	25. _____
Other – external influence	26. _____
Other – family of origin	27. _____

Representation of others _____

1 Representations of others reflect a stable and integrated sense others as unique individuals, and a realistic view of others' view of the subject
2 Representations of others characterized by a clear reflective picture of the other that is integrated and relatively stable though may be somewhat superficial; demonstrates defensive distortion or instability of sense of others' view of subject (e.g., failure to appreciate that others view subject as successful or admirable)
3 Representations of others characterized by a clear reflective picture of the major attributes of the other; however, representations of others are unstable and/or superficial, may be self-referential; distorted / unclear view of how the respondent is seen by others
4 Superficial and/or unstable representations of others, but with ability to give a rudimentary (albeit contradictory and unstable or highly superficial) description of some external objects
5 Superficial and chaotic representations of others that is largely defined by the subject's anxieties, defenses and needs

OVERALL RATING OF IDENTITY _____

1 Consolidated identity
2 Consolidated Identity, but with some areas of slight deficit (e.g., very mild superficiality or instability in sense of self and/or representations of others)
3 Unstable sense of identity; some areas of stability coupled with areas of significant deficit
4 Moderate Identity diffusion – few areas of stability in sense of self and others; multiple, significant areas of deficit
5 Severe identity diffusion – no areas of stability in sense of self, highly contradictory, chaotically shifting views of self and others, inability to invest

OBJECT RELATIONS

Interpersonal relationships

Interpersonal relations - social isolation	28. _____
Interpersonal relations – problems / volatility	29. _____
Interpersonal relations – response to stress	30. _____
Interpersonal relations – temporal stability	31. _____
Interpersonal relations - at work / school – conflict	32. _____

Interpersonal relationships _____

1 Has at least one or more good friendships; duration of at least two years; consistent contact with closest friends; depth of involvement and investment; absence of significant conflict across most relationships
2 Some investment in one or more friendships; good relationship quality in at least one relationship, but may be more variable, superficial, and less invested than as described in #1 above; may be some variability in contact or disclosure with closest friends; minimal conflict in friendships and in workplace
3 Some seeking out of a number of more superficial friendships, either of shorter duration, significantly diminished intimacy, or lack of reciprocal disclosure; relationships may be stable but infused with aggression and conflict, either in friendships or workplace
4 Some acquaintances, few if any friends; relationships are impoverished and superficial or perhaps ridden with significant conflict across multiple settings
5 Absence of friends; description of friendships is entirely superficial; chaotic, conflict ridden relationships across multiple settings

Intimate Relationships and Sexuality

Intimate relations – history of	33. _____
Intimate relations – intimacy / interdependence	34. _____
Intimate relations – relationship economics	35. _____
Intimate relations – bored	36. _____
Intimate relations – sexual activity	37. _____
Intimate relations – sexual inhibition	38. _____
Intimate relations – sensuality	39. _____
Intimate relations – love and sex	40. _____

Intimate and Sexual Relationships _____

1 Presence of satisfying, intimate relations involving interdependence; able to combine love and sexuality in relationships with significant duration (i.e., longer than 6 months)
2 Presence of intimate relationships, but flawed / conflicted (e.g., inhibited, stormy, may be limited in terms of disclosure and intimacy); may report having loving attachments while being sexually inhibited with relationship partners; may report difficulty integrating sex and love
3 Intimacy limited by conflicts (e.g., dependency and vulnerability), may report trouble sustaining intimate relationships; relationships described are conflicted, relatively brief, and/or highly superficial; may report stable, longer term relationships characterized by severe inhibitions of sexuality and intimacy
4 Superficial, non-invested, brief attempts at intimacy and/or the inability to experience sensual aspects of sexuality; may have little sensual pleasure and/or pervasive invasion of aggression
5 Absence of intimate relations and no sexual activity

Internal Working Model of Relationships

Empathy	41. _____
Entitlement – 1	42. _____
Entitlement – 2	43. _____
Object constancy	44. _____
Need fulfilling 1 – association value	45. _____
Need fulfilling 2 – relationship economics	46. _____
Need fulfilling 3 – bored with others	47. _____

Internal working model of relationships _____

1 Does not view relationships in terms of need fulfillment; easily and consistently empathizes with the other's needs independent of those of the subject; easily sustains enduring interest in others over time
2 Does not generally think of the relationship in terms of need fulfillment, i.e., may think about what he/she is getting out of a relationship but this is not the central motivator for most relationships; empathizes with the other's needs independent of those of the subject, but not all the time or in all settings; able to sustain enduring interest in others over time
3 Tends to view relationships in terms of need-fulfillment; somewhat limited capacity for empathy with the other's needs independent of those of the subject and/or some impairment in capacity to sustain enduring interest over time
4 Sees relationships largely in terms of need fulfillment; capacity to empathize with the other's needs independent of the subject is severely impaired; has little capacity to sustain interest in others over time
5 Sees relationships entirely in terms of need fulfillment; no capacity to empathize with the other's needs independent of the subject; no capacity for interest in others

OVERALL RATING OF QUALITY OF OBJECT RELATIONS _____

1 Strong, durable, realistic, nuanced, satisfying object relations; relationships not seen in terms of need fulfillment, able to combine sexuality and intimacy
2 Attachments are generally strong and durable, but may be less so than in #1 above; similar to # 1 across dimensions of need fulfillment; some degree of impairment in intimate / sexual relationships
3 Attachments are present, but increasingly superficial, brittle, and flawed; increasing tendency to view relationships in terms of need fulfillment; limited capacity for empathy with the other's needs independent of those of the subject
4 Attachments are few and flawed; may see relationships largely in terms of need fulfillment; relationships may be highly superficial, with little capacity for empathy with the other's needs independent of those of the subject
5 Severe paucity of attachments; sees relationships entirely in terms of need fulfillment; no capacity for empathy; no capacity to sustain interest in others

PRIMITIVE DEFENSES

Paranoia	48. _____
Erratic behaviour	49. _____
Idealization / devaluation	50. _____
View of most important relationships	51. _____
Black and white thinking	52. _____
Primitive denial	53. _____
Externalization	54. _____
Projective identification	55. _____
Fantasy	56. _____
Somatization	57. _____

Primitive Defenses _____

1 No evidence that primitive defenses are employed
2 Some endorsement of primitive defenses, with clearly elaborated examples in at least some cases; clearly NOT the predominant defensive style of the respondent; may be limited to idealization / devaluation
3 Mixed pattern of endorsement of primitive defenses; shifts in perception of self and others are not pronounced, limited impairment in functioning due to use of primitive defenses
4 Consistent endorsement of primitive defenses, shifts in perception of self and others are relatively severe and pervasive; clear evidence of impairment in respondent's life due to these defense patterns
5 Pervasive use of primitive defenses (externalization, primitive denial, idealization, devaluation and splitting) , across situations, severe, radical shifts in perception of self and others to a degree that grossly interferes with functioning, richly elaborated examples

COPING / RIGIDITY

Anticipation	58. _____
Suppression	59. _____
Flexibility	60. _____
Self-blame	61. _____
Proactive coping	62. _____
Perfectionism	63. _____
Multi-tasking / shifting sets	64. _____
Control	65. _____
Worrying	66. _____
Challenges	67. _____

Coping / rigidity _____

1 Flexible, adaptive coping; stress resilience in most areas
2 Evidence of adaptive coping strategies; strategies are used, however, with less consistency or efficacy, or in some areas but not others; largely resilient to stress
3 Inconsistent in capacity for use of adaptive coping strategies, with subsequent vulnerability to stress; rigid coping
4 Few examples in which the use of adaptive coping strategies in response to either larger scale stressors or daily hassles, are demonstrated; rigid, maladaptive coping
5 Pervasively inflexible, maladaptive coping

AGGRESSION

Self-directed Aggression

Self neglect	68. _____
Risky behaviour	69. _____
Relief	70. _____
Suicidality	71. _____
Sexual excitement	72. _____

Self -directed Aggression ______

1 No, or extremely minor self -directed aggression, e.g., minor cuticle biting
2 Neglect of own health, but concerning relatively minor issues; or minor self–destructive behaviour e.g., more consistent, steady cuticle biting
3 Neglect of own health with potentially serious consequences
4 Non-lethal attacks on own body
5 One or more lethal attacks on own body

Other-directed Aggression

Temper	73. _____
Attacks on others – remorse	74. _____
Enjoyment of suffering of others	75. _____
Dangerous sex	76. _____
Threat of self-injury	77. _____
Intimidation	78. _____
Hatred	79. _____

Other-directed Aggression _____

1 Control, modulation, and integration of anger and aggression
2 Loss of control with verbal aggression; followed by guilt and reparation of relationship
3 Loss of control w. verbal aggression; some pleasure in controlling and intimidating others
4 Hatred with no physical attack; vicious verbal attack; sadistic control of others, e.g., through intimidation, threats to self
5 Hatred, physical attack intended to harm

OVERALL RATING OF AGGRESSION _____

1 Control, modulation and integration of anger and aggression; may include episodes of anger and verbal aggression but these appear to be appropriate to the situation
2 Aggression expressed through self -neglect, minor self -destructive behaviors, controlling interpersonal style; verbal aggression is more frequent and/or hostile
3 Aggressive behaviors may be predominantly self -directed; occasional tantrums, hostile verbal aggression; more episodic and less chronic and less severe and dangerous than in 4 and 5, below
4 Aggressive behaviors directed against others either with or without aggression towards self; may be characterized by self -directed aggression that is severe to lethal; aggression is somewhat less pervasive, chronic (i.e., more episodic) and less life-threatening than in #5; frequent tantrums, frequent episodes involving hostile verbal aggression
5 Aggressive behaviors pose a serious danger to the safety of others and/or self; pervasive tendencies towards severe, dangerous aggression with pleasure in hurting and/or controlling others

MORAL VALUES

Internalized moral values	80. _____
Questionable opportunities	81. _____
Moral struggle	82. _____
Lying / deceit	83. _____
Illegal activity	84. _____
Guilt	85. _____
Exploitation	86. _____
Sadism	87. _____

OVERALL RATING OF MORAL VALUES _____

1 No evidence of amoral or immoral behavior; mature and appropriate sense of concern and responsibility for potentially hurtful or unethical behavior; experiences guilt; internal moral compass is autonomous, consistent and flexible; no exploitation of others for personal gain

2 No antisocial behavior; some evidence of inconsequential immoral behavioral (e.g., lying, cheating); internal moral compass is autonomous and consistent, with some conflict/ambiguity involving questionable opportunities for personal gain; experiences guilt, but in such a way that ruminative self-recrimination is more prevalent than proactive efforts to make amends

3 Some unethical/immoral behavior, e.g., plagiarism, cheating, lying, white collar crime, minor shoplifting, no confrontation of victim; difficulty taking full responsibility for behaviors that are hurtful to others; some sense of internal moral standards, but considerable difficulty using these standards to guide behaviors

4 Presence of violent, aggressive antisocial behavior such as stealing from others; may involve, confrontation of victims, but absence of assault and generally absent of premeditation; moral orientation is towards not getting caught; little conflict around making use of questionable opportunities for personal gain at the expense of others; moral values and internal standards are inconsistent and corrupt; little sense of guilt / remorse

5 Presence of violent, aggressive antisocial behavior (assault, battery, premeditation); no comprehension of the notion of moral values; no sense of guilt / remorse; psychopathy

REALITY TESTING AND PERCEPTUAL DISTORTIONS

Reality testing – Paranoia	88. _____
Reality testing – overreaction	89. _____
Dissociation	90. _____
Depersonalization	91. _____
Bizarre thoughts / ideas	92. _____
Hallucinatory experiences	93. _____
Referential thinking	94. _____

REALITY TESTING AND PERCEPTUAL DISTORTIONS _____

1 No perceptual distortions, no disturbance in reality testing; does not feel or appear strange or different

2 Mild perceptual distortions (e.g., mild depersonalization, "feeling" fat or ugly) with intact reality testing; may feel different than others but accurately perceives that he / she does not appear strange to others

3 Moderate perceptual distortions (e.g., frequently hearing one's name, frequent somatization or feelings of depersonalization or derealization, gross distortion of body image) with largely intact reality testing; may exhibit paranoia, innocuous eccentricity, i.e., sense of being strange or different but typically does not appear so

4 Marked perceptual distortions (e.g., seeing one's face "melt" in the mirror) with variable reality testing; may experience more severe paranoia and/or eccentricity, i.e., sense of being bizarre, strange or different and at times appears so to others, including interviewer

5 Severe perceptual distortions (e.g., somatic delusions or hearing voices) with marked disturbance in reality testing; appears highly bizarre / strange to others, including interviewer

3 References

Abraham, K. (1921). Psycho-analytic studies on character-formation. In *Selected Papers on Psycho-Analysis.* (pp. 370-417). London: Hogarth Press, 1927.

Akhtar, S. (1992). *Broken Structures: Severe Personality Disorders and Their Treatment.* New York: Jason Aronson.

Aldenderfer, M. S. & Blashfield, R. K. (1984). *Cluster Analysis.* Thousand Oaks, CA: Sage Publications, Quantitative Applications in the Social Sciences Series No. 44.

American Psychiatric Association (1952). *Diagnostic and Statistical Manual of Mental Disorders.* Washington, DC: Author.

American Psychiatric Association (1987). *Diagnostic and Statistical Manual of Mental Disorders (3rd ed., rev.).* Washington, DC: Author.

American Psychiatric Association (1994). *Diagnostic and Statistical Manual of Mental Disorders (4th ed.).* Washington, DC: Author.

Arbeitskreis OPD (1996). *Operationalisierte Psychodynamische Diagnostik (OPD-1).* Bern: Verlag Hans Huber.

Arbeitskreis OPD (2006). *Operationalisierte Psychodynamische Diagnostik (OPD-2).* Bern: Verlag Hans Huber.

Argelander, H. (1970). *Das Erstinterview in der Psychotherapie.* Darmstadt: Wissenschaftliche Buchgesellschaft.

Backhaus, K., Erichson, B., Plinke, W., & Weiber, R. (2003). *Multivariate Analyseverfahren.* Berlin: Springer.

Balint, M. & Balint, E. (1961). *Psychotherapeutic Techniques in Medicine.* London: Tavistock Publications.

Bateman, A. & Fonagy, P. (1999). Effectiveness of partial hospitalization in the treatment of borderline personality disorder: a randomized controlled trial. *American Journal of Psychiatry, 156,* 1563-1569.

Bateman, A. W. & Fonagy, P. (2004a). Mentalization-based treatment of BPD. *Journal of Personality Disorders, 18,* 36-51.

Bateman, A. W. & Fonagy, P. (2004b). *Psychotherapy for borderline personality disorder: mentalization based treatment.* Oxford: Oxford University Press.

Bender, D. S., Dolan, R. T., Skodol, A. E., Sanislow, C. A., Dyck, I. R., McGlashan, T. H., Shea, M. T., Zanarini, M. C., Oldham, J. M., & Gunderson, J. G. (2001). Treatment utilization by patients with personality disorders. *American Journal of Psychiatry, 158,* 295-302.

Benjamin, L. S. (1974). Structural analysis of social behavior. *Psychological Review, 81,* 392-425.

Benjamin, L. S. (1993). Dimensional, Categorical, or Hybrid Analyses of Personality: A Response to Widiger's Proposal. *Psychological Inquiry, 4,* 91-134.

Benjamin, L. S. (1994a). The bridge is supposed to reach the clinic, not just another corner of the academy. *Psychological Inquiry, 5,* 336-343.

Benjamin, L. S. (1994b). SASB: A bridge between personality theory and clinical psychology. *Psychological Inquiry, 5,* 273-316.

Blashfield, R. K. & McElroy, R. A. (1987). The 1985 journal literature on the personality disorders. *Comprehensive Psychiatry, 28,* 536-546.

Blatt, S. J. (2007). (in press). A fundamental polarity in psychoanalysis: Implications for personality development, psychopathology, and the therapeutic process. Psychonanalytic Inquiry.

Blatt, S. J. & Shichman, S. (1983). Two primary configurations of psychopathology. *Psychoanal.Contemp.Thought, 6,* 187-254.

Block, J. (1995). A contrarian view of the five-factor approach to personality description. *Psychological Bulletin, 117,* 187-215.

Buchheim, P., Cierpka, M., Kächele, H., & Jimenez, P. (1987). Das „Strukturelle Interview" - ein Beitrag zur Integration von Psychopathologie und Psychodynamik im psychiatrischen Erstgespräch. *Fundamenta psychiatrica, 1,* 154-161.

Buss, A. H. & Durkee, A. (1957). An Inventory for Assessing Different Kinds of Hostility. *Journal of Consulting Psychology, 21,* 343-349.

Caligor, E., Kernberg, O. F., & Clarkin, J. F. (2007). *Handbook of Dynamic Psychotherapy for Higher Level Personality Pathology.* Washington, D.C.: American Psychiatric Publishing Inc.

Cantor, N., Smith, E. E., French, R. S., & Mezzich, J. (1980). Psychiatric diagnosis as prototype categorization. *Journal of Abnormal Psychology, 89,* 181-193.

Cierpka, M., Grande, T., Rudolf, G., von der Tann, M., Stasch, M., & and the OPD Task Force (2007). The Operationalized Psychodynamic Diagnostics System: Clinical Relevance, Reliability and Validity. *Psychopathology, 40,* 209-220.

Cierpka, M., Grande, T., Stasch, M., Oberbracht, C., Schneider, W., Schüssler, G., Heuft, G., Dahlbender, R. W., Schauenburg, H., & Schneider, G. (2001). Zur Validität der Operationalisierten Psychodynamischen Diagnostik (OPD). *Psychotherapeut, 46,* 122-133.

Clark, L. A. (1993). Manual for the Schedule for Nonadaptive and Adaptive Personality (SNAP). Minneapolis: University of Minnesota Press.

Clark, L. A., McEwen, J. L., Collard, L. M., & Hickok, G. (1993). Symptoms and traits of personality disorder: Two new methods for their assessment. *Psychological Assessment, 5,* 81-91.

Clark, L. A., Livesley, W. J., Schroeder, M. L., & Irish, S. (1996). The structure of maladaptive personality traits: Convergent validity between two systems. *Psychological Assessment, 8,* 294-303.

Clark, L. A., Simms, L. J., Wu, K. D., & Casillas, A. (2005). Manual for the Schedule for Nonadaptive and Adaptive Personality, Second Edition (SNAP-2). Minneapolis, MN: University of Minnesota Press.

Clarkin, J. F. (2003). *Making patient assessment meaningful: A comparison of the structural interview and the OPD.* Unpublished Manuscript.

Clarkin, J. F. & Lenzenweger, M. F. (2005). *Major theories of personality disorder (2nd ed).* New York: Guilford.

Clarkin, J.F., Kernberg, O.F., & Somavia, J. (1998). Assessment of the patient with borderline personality disorder for psychodynamic treatment. In: J.W. Barron (Ed.), *Making diagnosis meaningful: Enhancing evaluations and treatment of psychological disorders.* (pp. 299-318). Washington, D.C.: American Psychological Association.

Clarkin, J. F., Foelsch, P., & Kernberg, O. F. (2001). *The Inventory of Personality Organization.* White Plains, New York: The New York Hospital - Cornell Medical Center.

Clarkin, J. F., Yeomans, F., & Kernberg, O. F. (1999). *Psychotherapy of Borderline Personality.* New York: Wiley.

Clarkin, J. F., Yeomans, F. E., & Kernberg, O. F. (2006). *Psychotherapy for Borderline Personality: Focusing on Object Relations.* Washington, D.C.: American Psychiatric Publishing, Inc.

Clarkin, J. F., Hull, J. W., Cantor, J., & Sanderson, C. (1993). Borderline personality disorder and personality traits: A comparison of SCID-II BPD and NEO-PI. *Psychological Assessment, 5,* 472-476.

Clarkin, J. F., Caligor, E., Stern, B. L., & Kernberg, O. F. (2004). *Structured Interview of Personality Organization (STIPO). Unpublished Manuscript.* Personality Disorders Institute, Weill Medical College of Cornell University, New York. (Deutsche Übersetzung von S.Doering, Universität Münster).

Clarkin, J. F., Levy, K. N., Lenzenweger, M. F., & Kernberg, O. F. (2007). Evaluating three treatments for borderline personality disorder: A Multiwave Study. *American Journal of Psychiatry, 164,* 922-928.

Clarkin, J. F., Widiger, T. A., Frances, A., Hurt, S. W., & Gilmore, M. (1983). Prototypic typology and the borderline personality disorder. *Journal of Abnormal Psychology, 92,* 263-275.

Clarkin, J. F., Foelsch, P. A., Levy, K. N., Hull, J. W., Delaney, J. C., & Kernberg, O. F. (2001). The development of a psychodynamic treatment for patients with borderline personality disorder: a preliminary study of behavioral change. *Journal of Personality Disorders, 15,* 487-495.

Cleckley, H. (1941). *The Mask of Sanity: An attempt to clarify some issues about the socalled psychopathic personality.* St. Louis: Mosby. (5th ed. (1976)).

Costa, P. T. & McCrae, R. (1990). Personality disorders and the five-factor model of personality. *Journal of Personality Disorders, 4,* 362-371.

Costa, P. T. & McCrae, R. (1992a). The Five-Factor Model of Personality and its relevance to personality disorders. *Journal of Personality Disorders, 6,* 343-359.

Costa, P. T. & McCrae, R. R. (1992b). *Revised NEO Personality Inventory (NEO-PI-R) and NEO Five-Factor-Inventory (NEO-FFI) professional manual.* Odessa, FL: Psychological Assessment Ressources.

Costa, P. T. & McCrae, R. (1995). Domains and facets: Hierarchical personality assessment using the Revised NEO Personality Inventory. *Journal of Personality Assessment, 64,* 21-50.

Dahlbender, R. W., Buchheim, A., & Doering, S. (2004). OPD und AAI - Integrative Diagnostik von Struktur, Konflikt und Bindungsrepräsentation. *Persönlichkeitsstörungen, 8,* 251-261.

Derogatis, L. R. (1993). *Brief Symptom Inventory (BSI). Administration, scoring, and procedures manual, third edition.* Minneapolis: National Computer Services.

Deutsch, H. (1942). Some forms of emotional disturbance and their relationship to schizophrenia. *Psychoanalytic Quarterly, 11,* 301-321.

Dolan-Sewell, R.T., Krueger, R.F., & Shea, M.T. (2001). Co-occurrence with syndrome disorders. In: W.J. Livesley (Ed.), *Handbook of personality disorders: Therory, research, and treatment.* (pp. 84-104). New York: The Guilford Press.

Dührssen, A. (1981). *Die biographische Anamnese unter tiefenpsychologischem Aspekt.* Göttingen: Verlag für Medizinische Psychologie im Verlag Vandenhoeck & Ruprecht.

Erikson, E.H. (1950). Growth and crises of the healthy personality. In *Identity and the Life Cycle* (pp. 50-100). New York: International Universities Press, 1959.

Erikson, E.H. (1956). The problem of ego identity. In *Identity and the Life Cycle* (pp. 104-164). New York: International Universities Press, 1959.

Ermann, M. (2004). *Psychosomatische Medizin und Psychotherapie. Ein Lehrbuch auf psychoanalytischer Grundlage.* (4., überarbeitete und erweiterte Auflage ed.) Stuttgart: Kohlhammer.

Fairbairn, W. D. (1952). *An Object-Relations Theory of the Personality.* New York: Basic Books.

Fenichel, O. (1945). *The psychoanalytic theory of neurosis.* New York: Norton.

First, M. B., Spitzer, R. L., Gibbon, M., & Williams, J. B. W. (1995a). The Structured Clinical Interview for DSM-III-R Personality Disorders (SCID-II), Part I: Description. *Journal of Personality Disorders, 9,* 83-91.

First, M. B., Spitzer, R. L., Gibbon, M., Williams, J. B. W., Davies, M., Borus, J., & et al (1995b). The Structured Clinical Interview for DSM-III-R Personality Disorders (SCID-II), Part II: Multi-site test-retest reliability study. *Journal of Personality Disorders, 9,* 92-104.

First, M. B., Spitzer, R. L., Gibbon, M., Williams, J. B. W., & Benjamin, L. B. (1996). *Structured Clinical Interview for DSM-IV Axis II Personality Disorders (SCID-II, version 2.0).* Biometrics Research Department, New York State Psychiatric Institute.

Foelsch, P., Clarkin, J. F., Kernberg, O. F., Somavia, J., Normandin, L., & Lenzenweger, M. F. (2000). *The Inventory of Personality Organization: Initial psychometric properties.* Unpublished manuscript.

Fonagy, P. & Target, M. (1997). Attachment and reflective function: their role in self-organization. *Development and Psychopathology, 9,* 679-700.

Fonagy, P., Target, M., & Gergely, G. (2000). Attachment and borderline personality disorder. A theory and some evidence. *Psychiatric Clinics of North America, 23,* 103-viii.

Fonagy, P., Target, M., Steele, H., & Steele, M. (1998). *Reflective-Functioning Manual for Application to Adult Attachment Interviews (Version 5.0)* . London, University College London, 1998.

Fonagy, P., Leigh, T., Steele, M., Steele, H., Kennedy, R., Mattoon, G., Target, M., & Gerber, A. (1996). The relation of attachment status, psychiatric classification, and response to psychotherapy. *J.Consult Clin.Psychol., 64,* 22-31.

Frances, A. (1980). The DSM-III personality disorders section: a commentary. *American Journal of Psychiatry, 137,* 1050-1054.

Freud, S. (1908). *Character and anal erotism. Standard Edition, 9: 167-175.* London: Hogarth Press, 1959.

Freud, S. (1923). *The ego and the id. Standard Edition, 19: 3-66.* London: Hogarth Press, 1961.

Freud, S. (1931). *Libidinal Types. Standard Edition, 21: 217-220.* London: Hogarth Press, 1961.

Fydrich, T. & Schmitz, B. (1996). Persönlichkeitsstörungen: Beiträge zur Diagnostik, Prävalenz und Validität. In: B. Schmitz, T. Fydrich, & K. Limbacher (Eds.), *Diagnostik und Psychotherapie bei Persönlichkeitsstörungen* - Weinheim: Beltz - Psychologie Verlags Union.

George, C., Kaplan, N., & Main, M. (1985). The Berkeley Adult Attachment Interview. Unpublished manuscript. Universtiy of Claifornia, Berkeley.

Grande, T., Rudolf, G., Oberbracht, C., & Jakobsen, T. (2001). [Therapeutic changes beyond the symptoms - effects of inpatient treatment according to the Heidelberg Structural Change Scale]. *Z.Psychosom.Med.Psychother., 47,* 213-233.

Grant, B. F., Hasin, D. S., Stinson, F. S., Dawson, D. A., Chou, S. P., Ruan, W. J., & Pickering, R. P. (2004). Prevalence, Correlates, and Disability of Personality Disorders in the United States: Results From the National Epidemiologic Survey on Alcohol and Related Conditions. *Journal of Clinical Psychiatry, 65,* 948-958.

Gross, R., Olfson, M., Gameroff, M., Shea, S., Feder, A., Fuentes, M., Lantigua, R., & Weissman, M. M. (2002). Borderline personality disorder in primary care. *Archives of Internal Medicine, 162,* 53-60.

Henderson, D. K. (1939). *Psychopathic States.* London: Chapman and Hall.

Herpertz, S., Steinmeyer, E. M., & Sass, H. (1994). "Patterns of comorbidity" among DSM-III-R and ICD-10 personality disorders as observed with a new inventory for the assessment of personality disorders. *European Archives of Psychiatry and Clinical Neuroscience, 244,* 161-169.

Hoerz, S., Stern, B. L., Caligor, E., Critchfield, K. L., Kernberg, O. F., Mertens, W., & Clarkin, J. F. (2007). What is prototypical of Borderline Personality Organization? Development of a prototypical profile based on the Structured Interview of Personality Organization (STIPO). Poster Presentation at the 38th Annual Meeting of the Society of Psychotherapy Research (SPR). Madison, 2007.

Hoffmann, S.O. (1998). Die Entwicklung einer Operationalisierten Psychodynamischen Diagnostik. In: H. Schauenburg, H.J. Freyberger, M. Cierpka, & P. Buchheim (Eds.), *OPD in der Praxis. Konzepte, Anwendungen, Ergebnisse der Operationalisierten Psychodynamischen Diagnostik.* (pp. 97-104). Bern: Hans Huber.

Horowitz, L. M., Rosenberg, S. E., Baer, B. A., Ureno, G., & Villasenor, V. S. (1988). Inventory of interpersonal problems: psychometric properties and clinical applications. *J.Consult Clin.Psychol., 56,* 885-892.

Huber, D., Klug, G., & Wallerstein, R. S. (2006). *Skalen Psychischer Kompetenzen (SPK). Ein Messinstrument für therapeutische Veränderung in der psychischen Struktur.* Stuttgart: Kohlhammer.

Jacobson, E. (1964). *The Self and the Object World.* New York: International Universities Press.

Jacobson, E. (1971). *Depression.* New York: International Universities Press.

John, O. P., Donahue, E. M., & Kentle, R. L. (1991). *The Big Five Inventory: Versions 4a and 54.* Technical report, Institute of Personality and Social Research, University of California, Berkeley, CA.

Johnson, C. & Wonderlich, S.A. (1992). Personality characteristics as a risk factor in the development of eating disorders. In: J.H. Crowther, D.L. Tennenbaum, S.E. Hobfoll, & M.A.P. Stephens (Eds.), *The Etiology of Bulimia Nervosa: The Individual and Familial Context.* - Washington, D.C.: Hemisphere Publishing Corp.

Kass, F., Skodol, A. E., Charles, E., Spitzer, R. L., & Williams, J. B. (1985). Scaled ratings of DSM-III personality disorders. *American Journal of Psychiatry, 142,* 627-630.

Kaye, A.L. & Shea, M.T. (2000). Personality disorders, personality traits, and defense mechanisms. In: Task Force for the Handbook of Psychiatric Measures (Ed.), *Handbook of Psychiatric Measures* (pp. 713-749). Washington, DC: American Psychiatric Association.

Kendall, R. (1982). The choice of diagnostic criteria for biological research. *Archives of General Psychiatry, 39,* 1334-1339.

Kernberg, O. F. (1975). *Borderline Conditions and Pathological Narcissism.* New York: Aronson.

Kernberg, O. F. (1976). *Object Relations Theory and Clinical Psychoanalysis.* New York: Jason Aronson.

Kernberg, O. F. (1980). *Internal World and External Reality: Object Relations Theory Applied.* New York: Jason Aronson.

Kernberg, O. F. (1981). Structural interviewing. *Psychiatric Clinics of North America, 4,* 169-195.

Kernberg, O. F. (1982). Self, ego, affects, and drives. *Journal of the American Psychoanalytic Association, 30,* 893-917.

Kernberg, O. F. (1984). *Severe personality disorders: Psychotherapeutic strategies.* New Haven, CT: Yale University Press.

Kernberg, O. F. (1992). *Aggression in personality disorders and perversions.* New Haven, CT: Yale University Press.

Kernberg, O.F. (1996). A psychoanalytic theory of personality disorders. In: J.F. Clarkin & M.F. Lenzenweger (Eds.), *Major theories of personality disorders* - New York: Guilford Press.

Kernberg, O.F. (1998). Die Bedeutung neuerer psychoanalytischer und psychodynamischer Konzepte für die Befunderhebung und Klassifikation von Persönlichkeitsstörungen. In: H. Schauenburg, H.J. Freyberger, & P. Buchheim (Eds.), *OPD in der Praxis. Konzepte, Anwendungen, Ergebnisse der Operationalisierten Psychodynamischen Diagnostik* - Bern: Verlag Hans Huber.

Kernberg, O.F. (2000). Borderlineorganisation und Klassifikation der Persönlichkeitsstörung. In: O.F. Kernberg, B. Dulz, & U. Sachsse (Eds.), (pp. 45-56). Stuttgart: Schattauer.

Kernberg, O. F. (2004). *Contemporary controversies in psychoanalytic theory, techniques and their application.* New Haven, CT: Yale University Press.

Kernberg, O.F. (2005). Psychoanalytic Object Relations Theories: Theory and Technique. In: E.S. Person, A.M. Cooper, & G.O. Gabbard (Eds.), *The American Psychiatric Publishing Textbook of Psychoanalysis* - Washington, DC: American Psychiatric Publishing.

Kernberg, O.F. & Caligor, E. (2005). A psychoanalytic theory of personality disorders. In: M.F. Lenzenweger & J.F. Clarkin (Eds.), *Major theories of personality disorder, second edition* (pp. 114-156). New York: Guilford Press.

Kim, Y., Pilkonis, P. A., & Barkham, M. (1997). Confirmatory factor analysis of the personality disorder subscales from the Inventory of Interpersonal Problems. *Journal of Personality Assessment, 69,* 284-296.

Klein, M. (1940). Mourning and its relation to manic-depressive states. In *Contributions to Psychoanalysis, 1921-1945* (pp. 311-338). London: Hogarths Press, 1948.

Klein, M. (1945). The Oedipus complex in the light of early anxieties. In *Contributions to Psychoanalysis, 1921-1945* (pp. 379-390). London: Hogarth press, 1948.

Klein, M. (1946). Notes on some schizoid mechanisms. *International Journal of Psychoanalysis, 27,* 99-110.

Klein, M. (1957). *Envy and Gratitude.* New York: Basic Books.

Koch, J. L. A. (1891). *The psychopathic inferiorities.* Ravensburg, Germany: Dorn.

Kohut, H. (1971). *The Analysis of the Self.* New York: International Universities Press.

Krueger, R. F. (1999). The structure of common mental disorders. *Archives of General Psychiatry, 56,* 921-926.

Lenzenweger, M. F., Clarkin, J. F., Kernberg, O. F., & Foelsch, P. A. (2001). The Inventory of Personality Organization: psychometric properties, factorial composition, and criterion relations with affect, aggressive dyscontrol, psychosis proneness, and self-domains in a nonclinical sample. *Psychological Assessment, 13,* 577-591.

Lenzenweger, M. F., Lane, M. C., Loranger, A. W., & Kessler, R. C. (2007). DSM-IV Personality Disorders in the National Comorbidity Survey Replication. *Biological Psychiatry.*

Levy, K. N., Meehan, K. B., Kelly, K. M., Reynoso, J. S., Weber, M., Clarkin, J. F., & Kernberg, O. F. (2006). Change in attachment patterns and reflective function in a randomized control trial of transference-focused psychotherapy for borderline personality disorder. *J.Consult Clin.Psychol., 74,* 1027-1040.

Linehan, M. M. (1993). *Cognitive-behavioural treatment of borderline personality disorder.* New York: Guilford.

Linehan, M. M., Schmidt, H., III, Dimeff, L. A., Craft, J. C., Kanter, J., & Comtois, K. A. (1999). Dialectical behavior therapy for patients with borderline personality disorder and drug-dependence. *American Journal on Addictions, 8,* 279-292.

Livesley, W. J. (1985). The classification of personality disorder: I. The choice of category concept. *Can.J.Psychiatry, 30,* 353-358.

Livesley, W. J. (1998). Suggestions for a framework for an empirically based classification of personality disorder. *Canadian Journal of Psychiatry, 43,* 137-147.

Livesley, W.J. (2003). Diagnostic dilemmas in classifying personality disorder. In: K.A. Phillips, M.B. First, & H.A. Pincus (Eds.), *Advancing DSM: Dilemmas in psychiatric diagnosis.* (pp. 153-190). Washington, D.C.: American Psychiatric Association.

Lohmer, M. (1988). *Stationäre Psychotherapie bei Borderline-Patienten.* Berlin, Heidelberg, New York: Springer.

Loranger, A. W. (1990). The impact of DSM-III on diagnostic practice in a university hospital. A comparison of DSM-II and DSM-III in 10,914 patients. *Archives of General Psychiatry, 47,* 672-675.

Loranger, A. W. (1999). *International Personality Disorder Examination (IPDE): DSM-IV and ICD-10 Modules.* Odessa, FL: Psychological Assessment Resources.

Loranger, A. W., Janca, A., & Sartorius, N. (1997). Assessment and diagnosis of personality disorders. The ICD-10 International Personality Disorder Examination (IPDE). Cambridge: Cambridge University Press.

Loranger, A. W., Sartorius, N., Andreoli, A., Berger, P., Buchheim, P., Channabasavanna, S. M., Coid, B., Dahl, A., Diekstra, R. F., Ferguson, B., & . (1994). The International Personality Disorder Examination. The World Health Organization/Alcohol, Drug Abuse, and Mental Health Administration international pilot study of personality disorders. *Archives of General Psychiatry, 51,* 215-224.

Luborsky, L. & Crits-Christoph, P. (1998). *Understanding Transference- The Core Conflictual Relationship Theme Method.* Washington, DC: American Psychological Association.

Lynam, D. R. & Widiger, T. A. (2001). Using the five-factor model to represent the DSM-IV personality disorders: an expert consensus approach. *Journal of Abnormal Psychology, 110,* 401-412.

Mahler, M. S. (1968). *On human symbiosis and the vicissitudes of individuation.* New York: International Universities Press.

Mahler, M. S., Pine, F., & Bergman, A. (1975). *The Psychological Birth of the Human Infant: Symbiosis and Individuation.* New York: Basic Books.

McGlashan, T. H., Grilo, C. M., Skodol, A. E., Gunderson, J. G., Shea, M. T., Morey, L. C., Zanarini, M. C., & Stout, R. L. (2000). The Collaborative Longitudinal Personality Disorders Study: baseline Axis I/II and II/II diagnostic co-occurrence. *Acta Psychiatrica Scandinavica, 102,* 256-264.

Melley, A. H., Oltmanns, T. F., & Turkheimer, E. (2002). The Schedule for Nonadaptive and Adaptive Personality (SNAP): Temporal Stability and Predictive Validity of the Diagnostic Scales. *Assessment, 9,* 181-187.

Mellsop, G., Varghese, F., Joshua, S., & Hicks, A. (1982). The reliability of axis II of DSM-III. *American Journal of Psychiatry, 139,* 1360-1361.

Merikangas, K.R. & Weissman, M.M. (1986). Epidemiology of *DSM-III* Axis II personality disorders. In: A.J. Francis & R.E. Hales (Eds.), *Psychiatric update: The*

American Psychiatric Association annual review (Vol. 5). - Washington, DC: American Psychiatric Press.

Mertens, W. (1992). *Einführung in die psychoanalytische Therapie, Band 1.* Stuttgart: Kohlhammer, 2. Auflage.

Mertens, W. (1993). *Einführung in die psychoanalytische Therapie. Band 2.* Stuttgart: Kohlhammer. 2. Auflage.

Mertens, W. & Waldvogel, B. (2002). *Handbuch psychoanalytischer Grundbegriffe.* Stuttgart: Kohlhammer, 2. Auflage.

Mestel, R., Klingelhöfer, J., Dahlbender, R.W., & Schüssler, G. (2004). Validität der OPD-Achsen Konflikt und Struktur in der stationären psychosomatischen Rehabilitation. In: R.W. Dahlbender, P. Buchheim, & G. Schüssler (Eds.), *Lernen an der Praxis. OPD und Qualitätssicherung in er Psychodynamischen Psychotherapie.* (pp. 229-244). Bern: Hans Huber.

Miller, J. D., Lynam, D. R., Widiger, T. A., & Leukefeld, C. (2001). Personality disorders as extreme variants of common personality dimensions: can the Five-Factor Model adequately represent psychopathy? *Journal of Personality, 69,* 253-276.

Moran, P., Rendu, A., Jenkins, R., Tylee, A., & Mann, A. (2001). The impact of personality disorder in UK primary care: a 1-year follow-up of attenders. *Psychological Medicine, 31,* 1447-1454.

Morey, L. C., Warner, M. B., Shea, M. T., Gunderson, J. G., Sanislow, C. A., Grilo, C., Skodol, A. E., & McGlashan, T. H. (2003). The representation of four personality disorders by the schedule for nonadaptive and adaptive personality dimensional model of personality. *Psychological Assessment, 15,* 326-332.

Noyes, R., Jr., Reich, J., Christiansen, J., Suelzer, M., Pfohl, B., & Coryell, W. A. (1990). Outcome of panic disorder. Relationship to diagnostic subtypes and comorbidity. *Archives of General Psychiatry, 47,* 809-818.

Nurnberg, H. G., Raskin, M., Levine, P. E., Pollack, S., Siegel, O., & Prince, R. (1991). The comorbidity of borderline personality disorder and other DSM-III-R axis II personality disorders. *American Journal of Psychiatry, 148,* 1371-1377.

Oldham, J. M., Skodol, A. E., Kellman, H. D., Hyler, S. E., Rosnick, L., & Davies, M. (1992). Diagnosis of DSM-III-R personality disorders by two structured interviews: patterns of comorbidity. *American Journal of Psychiatry, 149,* 213-220.

OPD Task Force (2001). *Operationalized Psychodynamic Diagnostics (OPD): Foundations and Manual.* Seattle: Hogrefe and Huber Publications.

Penna, M.W. (1981). Classification of personality disorders. In: J.R. Lion (Ed.), *Personality disorders. Diagnosis and management. (2nd ed., revised for DSM-III; pp. 10-31)* - Baltimore: Williams & Wilkins.

Perry, J. C., Banon, E., & Ianni, F. (1999). Effectiveness of psychotherapy for personality disorders. *American Journal of Psychiatry, 156,* 1312-1321.

Pfohl, B. (1999). Axis I and II: Comorbidity or confusion? In: C.R. Cloninger (Ed.), *Personality and psychopathology.* (pp. 83-98). Washington, D.C.: American Psychiatric Press.

Pfohl, B., Blum, N., & Zimmerman, M. (1997). *Structured Interview for DSM-IV Personality.* Washington, DC: American Psychiatric Press..

Pfohl, B., Blum, N., Zimmerman, M., & Stangl, D. (1989). Structured Interview for DSM-II-R Personality (SIDP-R). Iowa City: University of Iowa, Department of Psychiatry.

Pilkonis, P. A., Kim, Y., Proietti, J. M., & Barkham, M. (1996). Scales for personality disorders developed from the Inventory of Interpersonal Problems. *Journal of Personality Disorders, 10,* 335-369.

Pilkonis, P. A., Heape, C. L., Proietti, J. M., Clark, S. W., McDavid, J. D., & Pitts, T. E. (1995). The reliability and validity of two structured diagnostic interviews for personality disorders. *Archives of General Psychiatry, 52,* 1025-1033.

Pinel, P. (1809). *Traité médico-philosophique sur l'aliénation mentale. (2ieme edition).* Paris: Brosson.

Rabin, R. & de, C. F. (2001). EQ-5D: a measure of health status from the EuroQol Group. *Annals of Medicine, 33,* 337-343.

Reich, W. (1933). *Character Analysis.* New York: Noonday Press, 3rd edition, 1949.

Reich, J., Yates, W., & Nduaguba, M. (1989). Prevalence of DSM-III personality disorders in the community. *Social Psychiatry and Psychiatric Epidemiology, 24,* 12-16.

Rendu, A., Moran, P., Patel, A., Knapp, M., & Mann, A. (2002). Economic impact of personality disorders in UK primary care attenders. *British Journal of Psychiatry, 181,* 62-66.

Reynolds, S. K. & Clark, L. A. (2001). Predicting personality disorder dimensions from domains and facets of the five-factor model. *Journal of Personality, 69,* 199-222.

Rudolf, G., Oberbracht, C., & Grande, T. (1998). Die Struktur-Checkliste. Ein anwenderfreundliches Hilfsmittel für die Strukturdiagnostik nach OP. In: H. Schauenburg, H.J. Freyberger, M. Cierpka, & P. Buchheim (Eds.), *OPD in der Praxis. Konzepte, Anwendungen, Ergebnisse der Operationalisierten Psychodynamischen Diagnostik.* (pp. 167-181). Bern: Hans Huber.

Rudolf, G., Grande, T., Oberbracht, C., & Jacobsen, T. (1996). Erste empirische Untersuchungen zu einem neuen diagnostischen System: Die Operationalisierte Psychodynamische Diagnostik (OPD). *Zeitrschrift für Psychosomatische Medizin und Psychotherapie, 42,* 343-357.

Samuel, D. B. & Widiger, T. A. (2004). Clinicians' personality descriptions of prototypic personality disorders. *Journal of Personality Disorders, 18,* 286-308.

Sanislow, C. A., Morey, L. C., Grilo, C. M., Gunderson, J. G., Shea, M. T., Skodol, A. E., Stout, R. L., Zanarini, M. C., & McGlashan, T. H. (2002). Confirmatory factor analysis of DSM-IV borderline, schizotypal, avoidant and obsessive-compulsive personality disorders: findings from the Collaborative Longitudinal Personality Disorders Study. *Acta Psychiatrica Scandinavica, 105,* 28-36.

Sartorius, N., Kaelber, C. T., Cooper, J. E., Roper, M. T., Rae, D. S., Gulbinat, W., Ustun, T. B., & Regier, D. A. (1993). Progress toward achieving a common language in psychiatry. Results from the field trial of the clinical guidelines accompanying the WHO classification of mental and behavioral disorders in ICD-10. *Archives of General Psychiatry, 50,* 115-124.

Scarpa, A., Luscher, K. A., Smalley, K. J., Pilkonis, P. A., Kim, Y., & Williams, W. C. (1999). Screening for personality disorders in a nonclinical population. *Journal of Personality Disorders, 13,* 345-360.

Schauenburg, H., Janssen, P.L., & Buchheim, P. (1998). Interviewführung in der OPD. In: H. Schauenburg, H.J. Freyberger, M. Cierpka, & P. Buchheim (Eds.), *OPD in der Praxis. Konzepte, Anwendungen, Ergebnisse der Operationalisierten Psychodynamischen Diagnostik.* (pp. 139-158). Bern: Hans Huber.

Schneider, K. (1950). *Psychopathic personalities (9th ed.).* London: Cassell (original work published 1923).

Shearer, S. L. (1994). Phenomenology of self-injury among inpatient women with borderline personality disorder. *Journal of Nervous and Mental Disease, 182,* 524-526.

Shrout, P. E. & Fleiss, J. L. (1979). Intraclass correlations: Uses in assessing rater reliability. *Psychological Bulletin, 86,* 420-428.

Simms, L. J. & Clark, L. A. (2001). Detection of deception on the Schedule for Nonadaptive and Adaptive Personality: Validation of the validity scales. *Assessment, 8,* 251-266.

Skodol, A. E., Gunderson, J. G., Pfohl, B., Widiger, T. A., Livesley, W. J., & Siever, L. J. (2002). The borderline diagnosis I: psychopathology, comorbidity, and personality structure. *Biological Psychiatry, 51,* 936-950.

Skodol, A. E., Gunderson, J. G., Shea, M. T., McGlashan, T. H., Morey, L. C., Sanislow, C. A., Bender, D. S., Grilo, C. M., Zanarini, M. C., Yen, S., Pagano, M. E., & Stout, R. L. (2005). The Collaborative Longitudinal Personality Disorders Study (CLPS): overview and implications. *Journal of Personality Disorders, 19,* 487-504.

Soloff, P. H., Lis, J. A., Kelly, T., Cornelius, J., & Ulrich, R. (1994). Risk factors for suicidal behavior in borderline personality disorder. *American Journal of Psychiatry, 151,* 1316-1323.

Spitzer, C., Michels-Lucht, F., Siebel, U., & Freyberger, H. J. (2002). [The axis "Structure" of the operationalized psychodynamic diagnostics (OPD): Its relationship with sociodemographic, clinical and psychopathological features as well as categorical diagnoses]. *Psychotherapie, Psychosomatik, Medizinische Psychologie, 52,* 392-397.

Spitzer, R. L., Forman, J. B., & Nee, J. (1979). DSM-III field trials: I. Initial interrater diagnostic reliability. *American Journal of Psychiatry, 136,* 815-817.

Stasch, M., Cierpka, M., Hillenbrand, E., & Schmal, H. (2002). Assessing reenactment in inpatient psychodynamic therapy. *Psychotherapy Research, 2002,* 355-368.

Stern, B. L., Kim, Y., Trull, T. J., Scarpa, A., & Pilkonis, P. (2000). Inventory of Interpersonal Problems Personality Disorder scales: operating characteristics and confirmatory factor analysis in nonclinical samples. *Journal of Personality Assessment, 74,* 459-471.

Stern, B. L., Caligor, E., Roose, S. P., & Clarkin, J. F. (2004a). The Structured Interview for Personality Organization (STIPO): Reliability and Validity. Poster Presentation at the Winter Meeting of the American Psychoanalytic Association, New York City, January 2004.

Stern, B. L., Maccornack, V., Caligor, E., Hoerz, S., Cassab, J., Clarkin, J. F., & Kernberg, O. F. (2004b). The Structured Interview for Personality Organization (STIPO): Preliminary Reliability and Validity. Poster Presentation at the 35th Annual Meeting of the Society of Psychotherapy Research (SPR). Rome, 2004.

Stern, B. L., Caligor, E., Clarkin, J. F., Critchfield, K. L., Maccornack, V., & Kernberg, O. F. (2007). The Structured Interview of Personality Organization (STIPO): Preliminary Psychometrics in a Clinical Sample. (Under review).

Sullivan, H. S. (1954). *The Psychiatric Interview.* New York, London: Norton.

Torgersen, S., Kringlen, E., & Cramer, V. (2001). The prevalence of personality disorders in a community sample. *Archives of General Psychiatry, 58,* 590-596.

Trull, T. J., Widiger, T. A., Lynam, D. R., & Costa, P. T., Jr. (2003). Borderline personality disorder from the perspective of general personality functioning. *Journal of Abnormal Psychology, 112,* 193-202.

van Asselt, A. D., Dirksen, C. D., Arntz, A., & Severens, J. L. (2007). The cost of borderline personality disorder: societal cost of illness in BPD-patients. *Eur.Psychiatry.*

Verheul, R. & Widiger, T. A. (2004). A meta-analysis of the prevalence and usage of the personality disorder not otherwise specified (PDNOS) diagnosis. *Journal of Personality Disorders, 18,* 309-319.

Verheul, R., van den, B. W., & Hartgers, C. (1998). Personality disorders predict relapse in alcoholic patients. *Addictive Behaviors, 23,* 869-882.

Wallerstein, R.S. (1991). Assessment of structural change in psychoanalytic therapy and research. In: T. Shapiro (Ed.), *The concept of structure in psychoanalysis* (pp. 241-261). Madison: International University Press.

Ward, C., Beck, A., Mendelson, M., Mock J., & Erbaugh, J. (1962). The psychiatric nomenclature. Reasons for diagnostic disagreement. *Archives of General Psychiatry, 7,* 205.

Watson, D. C. & Sinha, B. K. (1998). Comorbidity of DSM-IV personality disorders in a nonclinical sample. *Journal of Clinical Psychology, 54,* 773-780.

Watson, D., Clark, L. A., & Harkness, A. R. (1994). Manual for the Positive and Negative Affect Schedule (Expanded Form).University of Iowa.

Watson, D., Clark, L. A., & Tellegen, A. (1988). Development and validation of brief measures of Positive and Negative Affect: The PANAS Scales. *Journal of Personality and Social Psychology, 54,* 1063-1070.

Weidenhammer, B. (1987). Störungen des diagnostischen Urteilsprozesses bei präödipalen Pathologien. [Disorders of the diagnostic judgment process in pre-oedipal pathologies]. *Zeitschrift für Psychosomatische Medizin und Psychoanalyse, 33,* 353-362.

Weinryb, R.M. (1998). Zur Diagnose der Charakterstruktur mit dem "Karolinska Psychodynamic Profile" (KAPP). In: H. Schauenburg, H.J. Freyberger, M. Cierpka, & P. Buchheim (Eds.), *OPD in der Praxis. Konzepte, Anwendungen, Ergebnisse der Operationalisierten Psychodynamischen Diagnostik* (pp. 69-95). Bern: Hans Huber.

Weinryb, R. M. & Rossel, R. J. (1991). Karolinska Psychodynamic Profile. KAPP. *Acta Psychiatr.Scand.Suppl, 363,* 1-23.

Weinryb, R. M., Rossel, R. J., & Asberg, M. (1991b). The Karolinska Psychodynamic Profile. II. Interdisciplinary and cross-cultural reliability. *Acta Psychiatrica Scandinavica, 83,* 73-76.

Weinryb, R. M., Rossel, R. J., & Asberg, M. (1991a). The Karolinska Psychodynamic Profile. I. Validity and dimensionality. *Acta Psychiatrica Scandinavica, 83,* 64-72.

Weinryb, R. M., Gustavsson, J. P., Asberg, M., & Rossel, R. J. (1992). The concept of alexithymia: an empirical study using psychodynamic ratings and self-reports. *Acta Psychiatrica Scandinavica, 85,* 153-162.

Weinryb, R. M., Busch, M., Gustavsson, J. P., Saxon, L., & Skarbrandt, E. (1998). Reliability of the Karolinska Psychodynamic Profile (KAPP) among patients with and without psychoactive substance abuse disorders. *Psychotherapy and Psychosomatics, 67,* 10-16.

Westen, D. (1995). A clinical-empirical model of personality: life after the Mischelian ice age and the NEO-lithic era. *Journal of Personality, 63,* 495-524.

Westen, D. (1997). Divergences between clinical and research methods for assessing personality disorders: implications for research and the evolution of axis II. *Am.J.Psychiatry, 154,* 895-903.

Westen, D. & Shedler, J. (1999a). Revising and assessing axis II, Part I: developing a clinically and empirically valid assessment method. *American Journal of Psychiatry, 156,* 258-272.

Westen, D. & Shedler, J. (1999b). Revising and assessing axis II, Part II: toward an empirically based and clinically useful classification of personality disorders. *American Journal of Psychiatry, 156,* 273-285.

Westen, D. & Shedler, J. (2000). A prototype matching approach to diagnosing personality disorders: toward DSM-V. *Journal of Personality Disorders, 14,* 109-126.

Westen, D., Gabbard, G.O., & Blagov, P. (2006). Back to the future: Personality structure as a context for psychopathology. In: R.F. Krueger & J.L. Tackett (Eds.), *Personality and psychopathology.* - New York: Guilford.

Westen, D., Shedler, J., & Bradley, R. (2006). A prototype approach to personality disorder diagnosis. *American Journal of Psychiatry, 163,* 846-856.

Widiger, T. A. & Costa, P. T., Jr. (1994). Personality and personality disorders. *Journal of Abnormal Psychology, 103,* 78-91.

Widiger, T. A. & Frances, A. (1985). The DSM-III personality disorders. Perspectives from psychology. *Archives of General Psychiatry, 42,* 615-623.

Widiger, T.A. & Frances, A.J. (1989). Epidemiology, diagnosis, and comorbidity of borderline personality disorder. In: A. Tasman, R.E. Hales, & A.J. Frances (Eds.), *American Psychiatric Press Review of Psychiatry, Volume 8* (pp. 8-24). Washington, DC: American Psychiatric Press.

Widiger, T. A. & Seidlitz, L. (2002). Personality, psychopathology, and aging. *Journal of Research in Personality, 36,* 335-362.

Widiger, T. A. & Simonsen, E. (2005). Alternative dimensional models of personality disorder: finding a common ground. *Journal of Personality Disorders, 19,* 110-130.

Widiger, T. A., Hurt, S. W., Frances, A., Clarkin, J. F., & Gilmore, M. (1984). Diagnostic efficiency and DSM-III. *Archives of General Psychiatry, 41,* 1005-1012.

Widiger, T. A., Mangine, S., Corbitt, E. M., Ellis, C. G., & Thomas, G. V. (1995). *Personality Disorder Interview - IV: A Semi-structured Interview for the Assessment of Personality Disorders.* Odessa, FL.: Psychological Assessment Resources.

Widiger, T.A., Trull, T.J., Clarkin, J.F., Sanderson, C., & Costa, P.T. (1994). A description of the DSM-III-R and DSM-IV personality disorders with the five-factor model of personality. In: P.T. Costa & T.A. Widiger (Eds.), *Personality disorders and the five-factor model of personality.* (pp. 41-56). Washington, DC: American Psychological Association.

World Health Organization (1992). *International statistical classification of diseases and related health problems. (10th revision).* Geneva, Switzerland: Author.

Zanarini, M. C., Frankenburg, F. R., Chauncey, D. L., & Gunderson, J. G. (1987). The diagnostic Interview for Personality Disorders: interrater and test-retest reliability. *Comprehensive Psychiatry, 28,* 467-480.

Zanarini, M. C., Skodol, A. E., Bender, D., Dolan, R., Sanislow, C., Schaefer, E., Morey, L. C., Grilo, C. M., Shea, M. T., McGlashan, T. H., & Gunderson, J. G. (2000). The Collaborative Longitudinal Personality Disorders Study: reliability of axis I and II diagnoses. *Journal of Personality Disorders, 14,* 291-299.

Zimmerman, M. (1994). Diagnosing personality disorders. A review of issues and research methods. *Archives of General Psychiatry, 51,* 225-245.

Zimmerman, M., Coryell, W., & Black, D. W. (1993). A method to detect intercenter differences in the application of contemporary diagnostic criteria. *Journal of Nervous and Mental Disease, 181,* 130-134.

Zimmerman, M., Rothschild, L., & Chelminski, I. (2005). The prevalence of DSM-IV personality disorders in psychiatric outpatients. *American Journal of Psychiatry, 162,* 1911-1918.